FIRST AID TRAINING

FIRST ON THE SCENE
STUDENT REFERENCE GUIDE

Emergency First Aid for Industry with Alberta Endorsement

Recognition of injury -causing force

second edition 2006

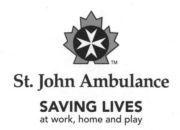

St. John Ambulance

SAVING LIVES
at work, home and play

www.sja.ca

Second Edition - 2006

St. John Ambulance
1900 City Park Drive, #400
Ottawa, Ontario
K1J 1A3

Library and Archives Canada Cataloguing in Publication

Main entry under title:
   First aid training: first on the scene. Student reference guide. — 1st ed.

Includes index.
First ed. published under title: First aid: first on the scene. Activity book.

ISBN 1-894070-56-9

   1. First aid in illness and injury—Problems, exercises, etc. 2. CPR
(First aid)—Problems, exercises, etc. I. St. John Ambulance

RC86.8.F598 2006   616.02'52   C2006-901820-0

Printed in Canada
Stock No. 6500-06

CONTENTS

Terms and Conditions of Certification

The first aid attendant must follow the principles of first aid treatment as outline in the WorkSafe BC OFA training programs.

The first aid certificate holder must not engage in inappropriate conduct, not restricted to but including:

* smoking while assessing or treating an injured or ill worker and/or while handling oxygen therapy equipment, or permitting others to do so;

* failure to use the assessment and injury treatment techniques outlined in first aid training courses unless conditions preclude them;

* conduct that poses an unreasonable threat to the safety and well-being of other workers or the public;

* removing themselves from being able to see or hear any summons for first aid at a workplace;

* abandonment of an injured worker after beginning assessment or treatment;

* refusal to treat an injured worker when acting as the designated attendant; or

* treating or transporting an injured worker while impaired or under the influence of drugs or alcohol

Contents

STUDENT INFORMATION

St. John Ambulance courses are nationally recognized standardized programs. They are based on performance objectives and well defined training standards which are contained in the Instructor's Guide for these courses.

This **student reference guide** is part of a sequenced training program, consisting of DVDsequences, instructor-led practical and activity book exercises.

Certification requirements

The training standards specify the minimum requirements for certification. Courses may be expanded, if necessary, to include additional material required to meet local needs.

To receive a certificate you must:

◆ attend the instructional sessions

◆ obtain a satisfactory pass on the practical exercises, and

◆ obtain a minimum mark of 70% on each section of the written examination

Your first aid certificate is valid for two years from the date the course was successfully completed.

Note: First aid skills deteriorate very quickly unless they are practised regularly. Recertification every two years in first aid is recommended.

USE OF THE STUDENT REFERENCE GUIDE

Please complete the Course Registration Form at the back of this book and hand it to your instructor.

On completion of the course, you will be asked to complete the Course Evaluation Form. This form is to be handed in to the Instructor before you leave the class on the final day.

Cardiovascular Emergencies - Activity

Angina and heart attack

1. _____ refers to disorders of the heart and blood vessels.
2. Narrowing of arteries is caused by a build up of _____ on the inside lining. This results in reduced _____ to the tissues on the other side of the narrowing.
3. _____ refers to the pain or discomfort in the chest which may spread to the neck, jaw, shoulders and arms. This pain does not last long and goes away if the person rests and takes prescribed medication.
4. Many people with angina live normally by taking _____ that increases blood flow to the heart.
5. A _____ happens when the heart muscle dies because its supply of oxygenated blood has been cut off.
6. Signs and symptoms of angina and heart attack include:
   a) _____
   b) _____
   c) _____
   d) _____
7. If you suspect someone is having a heart attack, it is important to get _____ right away.
8. If you suspect a casualty is having angina or a heart attack,
   a) place the casualty _____ to reduce the work of the heart.
   b) Help the casualty to take _____
   c) Give _____ if he loses consciousness and stops breathing.

4-1

Cardiovascular Emergencies - One Rescuer (CPR)

Welcome to the student reference guide exercises.

This reference guide will help you to learn the first aid theory for the course and will prepare you for the final written examination. Your instructor will tell you which exercises to complete and when to do them. Your Instructor may lead you through exercises as part of the theoretical program. Other exercises may be given to you to complete in self-study. Other exercises are provided for your reference and use but are not used in the formal presentation of the program.

ROLES AND DUTIES OF A FIRST AID ATTENDANT IN B.C.

To be prepared is essential . . .

The first aid attendant learns some basic procedures and steps so that an injured worker can be provided with adequate care while awaiting the arrival of medical help.

Preparedness means knowing about . . .

- the Occupational First Aid Regulations

- the operation and layout of the workplace

- specific hazardous substances and their first aid treatments – WHMIS

- specialized dangerous equipment and machinery and protocols for lockout

- transportation methods and access routes for their job site

- location of first aid equipment

- number of trained workers at their workplace, their availability and locations

- methods of communication for calling trained persons and getting available transportation to the injured worker

- need for specialized personnel and protective equipment

- the location of specialized personnel and protective equipment and ensuring its readiness at all times

- checklists that are available to ensure preparedness at the workplace

- Emergency Scene Management – a thorough step-by-step process to manage an injured worker efficiently and effectively.

TO BE PREPARED IS ESSENTIAL!

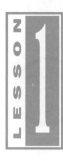

Objectives

- Apply the knowledge of terms used in first aid
- Apply the knowledge of legal implications when giving first aid
- Apply the principles of safety when giving first aid
- Apply the principles of first aid
- Apply the principles of emergency scene management
- Perform a scene survey
- Perform a primary survey
- Perform ongoing care until handover

What is first aid?

First aid is emergency help given to an injured or suddenly ill person using readily available materials. It can be simple, like removing a sliver from a child's finger and putting on a bandage, or it can be complicated, like giving care to many casualties in a motor vehicle collision and handing them over to medical help.

The objectives of first aid remain the same, regardless of the situation:

- preserve life
- prevent the illness or injury from becoming worse
- promote recovery

Who is a first aider?

A **first aider** is someone who takes charge of an emergency scene and gives first aid. First aiders don't *diagnose* or *treat* injuries or illnesses (except perhaps when they are very minor) - this is what medical doctors do. A first aider *suspects* injuries and illnesses and gives first aid.

The injured or ill person is called a **casualty.**

What can a first aider do?

Stand by, I might need your help!

A first aider gives first aid, but they can also do much more.

- protect the casualty's belongings
- keep unnecessary people away
- reassure family and friends of the casualty
- clean up the emergency scene and work to correct any unsafe conditions that may have caused the injury in the first place

First aid and the law

Can a first aider be sued for giving first aid? Fear of being sued is one of the main reasons why people don't help when help is needed most. As a first aider, there are two legal situations in which you might give first aid. First, you may give first aid as part of your job, for example, as a lifeguard, or first aid attendant. Second you might simply be a passer-by who sees an emergency situation and wishes to help an injured or ill person.

Giving first aid as part of your job

When giving first aid as part of your job, you have a legal duty to respond to an emergency situation at your workplace. You have a duty to use reasonable skill and care based on your level of training. This might include more than first aid - you may be trained in rescue, driving an emergency vehicle, etc. If you are a designated first aider at work, **make sure your certification is always up to date.** If you can, get a level of training higher than the minimum - you will be a more confident and effective first aider.

Giving first aid as a passer-by

In Canada (except Quebec) and most of the United States, you do not have a legal duty to help a person in need - if you do not help an injured person, you are not at fault. But our governments want to encourage people to help others, so they recognize the Good Samaritan Principles. These principles protect you if you choose to help someone in need. Once you begin to give assistance, you are obligated to use reasonable skill and care based on your level of training.

Giving first aid in Quebec

The *Quebec Charter of Human Rights and Freedoms* declares that any person whose life is in danger has the right to be helped. This means that you are required to help a person whose life is at risk, provided you do not put your own life, or anyone else's, in danger.

Principles of the Good Samaritan

You are a Good Samaritan if you help a person when you have no legal duty to do so. As a Good Samaritan, you give your help without being paid, and you give it in good faith (meaning you are helping because you care about the person and not for some other reason). Whenever you help a person in an emergency situation, you should abide by the following principles:

Consent - identify yourself as a first aider and get permission to help the injured or ill person before you touch her.

Reasonable skill and care - act according to the level of knowledge and skill you have.

Negligence - use common sense and make sure your actions are in the casualty's best interests

Abandonment - never abandon a casualty in your care. Stay with her until you hand her over to medical help, you hand her over to another first aider or she no longer wants your help. This is usually because the problem is no longer an emergency and further care is not needed.

Note that St. John Ambulance is not giving legal advice here. This information is not intended to replace advice given by a lawyer.

Safety and first aid

The number one rule in giving first aid is, "Give first aid safely." Emergency scenes can be dangerous and you have to make sure your actions don't put you or anyone else in danger. Take the time to look for hazards and assess the risks of any actions you take.

There are three basic types of risks to be aware of:

◆ the energy source that caused the original injury - is the energy still active and could anyone be injured by it? For example, where an injury has been caused by machinery, is the machinery still running?

◆ the hazards from external factors - are other conditions present that could be a hazard? For example, at the scene of a car crash, could there be an explosion or perhaps injuries caused by passing vehicles?

◆ the hazards of the rescue or first aid procedures - is there risk of someone being injured by the rescue and first aid actions? For example, if the casualty is much larger than you are, and you have to move that person, can you do so without injuring yourself?

Preventing infection

A first aider and casualty are in very close contact with each other when first aid is given. This close contact means that an infection could pass from one person to the other. This risk of infection is a safety hazard a first aider has to be aware of.

Some people are afraid to give first aid. They think they might catch a disease from the casualty, but people are most likely to be helping family and friends. The risk of a **serious** infection being transmitted is small but there are several types of disease you should be aware of when providing first aid.

Diseases caused by viruses and bacteria can be spread through the blood (bloodborne pathogens) or in the air through coughing or sneezing (airborne pathogens). There are many different types of diseases spread by either of these routes but a select few are of interest to first aiders.

Bloodborne Infections: There are 3 types of bloodborne disease that first aiders should be particularly aware of:

You can always do something

If you do not want to touch a casualty because of the risk of infection—is there anything you can do? Yes, there is plenty of first aid you can give. For instance, you can:

◆ take charge
◆ call bystanders and ask for help
◆ make the area safe
◆ send/get medical help
◆ give reassurance
◆ give information to ambulance officers

The risk of infection to a first aider is extremely small. In a situation where you think the risk is high, there are still many potentially life-saving actions you can take.

1. Human immunodeficiency virus (HIV). This virus is responsible for AIDs which affects the body's immune system and its ability to fight other diseases. Currently no vaccine exists to protect people from this virus and the best defense remains adequate protection to help prevent infection.

2. Hepatitis B. Hepatitis is a viral disease of the liver that can cause severe liver damage or liver cancer. There are 3 common forms of hepatitis - Type A, Type B and Type C depending on the type of virus causing the disease. Health care workers are at high risk for contacting this disease as are others involved in first response such as police officers, firefighters etc. Some people who have hepatitis B have no symptoms but can still have the virus in their blood and are therefore contagious. Fortunately a vaccine does exist that will prevent hepatitis B from occuring and the vaccine is usually made available to high risk individuals.

3. Hepatitis C. Hepatitis C causes much the same liver damage as hepatitis B but there is currently no vaccine available to prevent this disease

Airborne Infections. A number of diseases can be spread through the air usually by a person inhaling droplets when an infected person coughs or sneezes. The common cold is a good example but more serious diseases such as tuberculosis are also spread in this fashion.

There is more risk of serious infection when blood and other body fluids are involved, as the viruses that cause AIDS (acquired immunodeficiency syndrome), hepatitis B and other illnesses may be present. You should always use safety measures called *universal precautions* to minimize the risk of transmission.

Universal precautions are used in the health care professions to reduce the risk of infection for both the caregiver and the casualty. Universal precautions that apply to first aiders are:

◆ Gloves - wear gloves to prevent direct hand contact between the first aider and the casualty. Wear gloves when you might touch blood, body fluids or tissue

◆ Face masks or shield - use a face mask or shield designed to prevent disease transmission when providing artificial respiration or CPR. Follow the manufacturer's instructions on how to use, care for and dispose of a mask and shield properly

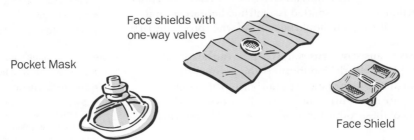

Face shields with one-way valves

Pocket Mask

Face Shield

◆ Hand washing - wash hands with soap and running water immediately after any contact with a casualty

If you have to clean up a blood spill use personal protection such as gloves. Wipe up the spill using paper towels or other absorbent material. After you have cleaned up the area cover it with a bleach solution (1/4 cup bleach (62.5mL) to 1 gallon (4 litres) of water) and let stand for at least 20 minutes. Cleaning materials contaminated with blood or other body fluids should be discarded in appropriate containers.

Clothing that has been stained with blood or vomitus should be thoroughly washed in a washing machine in hot water.

How to remove Gloves

Once gloves have been used, they are contaminated and are a possible source of infection. Take them off without touching their outer surface following the steps below.

1

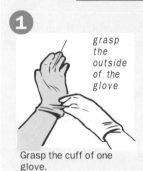

grasp the outside of the glove

Grasp the cuff of one glove.

2

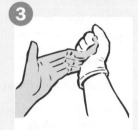

Pull the cuff towards the fingers, turning the glove inside out.

3

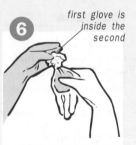

As the glove comes off, hold it in the palm of your other hand.

4

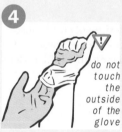

do not touch the outside of the glove

Slide your fingers under the cuff of the other glove.

5

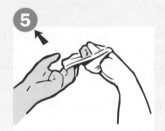

Pull the cuff towards the fingers over the first glove.

6

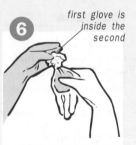

first glove is inside the second

Tie a knot in the top of the outer glove and dispose of properly—see below.

7

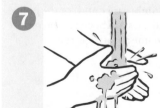

Wash hands with soap and running water as soon as possible.

Torn gloves

If you tear your gloves while giving first aid, take them off right away. Wash your hands if possible, and put on a new pair of gloves.

Proper disposal

Seal the used gloves in a plastic bag and put them in your household garbage.

Check with a health professional or your first aid instructor for specific regulations in your area.

Safety in a violent situation

Violent situations are not uncommon. Often there are injuries and your skills as a first aider can be valuable. In any emergency scene, be on the lookout for violence. If there is violence, or the potential for violence, be careful. Your first priority is to protect your own safety - don't put yourself at risk. You are more valuable as a first aider than as a casualty.

Whenever injuries occur through violence, a crime has been committed. If you think a crime has been committed, call the police to the scene. While waiting for the police:

- ◆ protect your safety, and the safety of others if you can

- ◆ give first aid for any injuries, and be sensitive to the casualty's emotional state

- ◆ keep onlookers away as much as possible - do what you can to ensure the privacy of any casualties

- ◆ leave everything at the scene as is - you may disturb evidence that could help the police in their investigation

As a first aider you may have other information the police will find helpful. Stay on the scene until the police say you can leave.

Child abuse

When giving first aid to a child with injuries, be on the alert for signs of child abuse. Child abuse is any form of physical harm, emotional deprivation, neglect or sexual maltreatment which can result in injury or psychological damage to the child. To detect possible child abuse, look for signs including:

- ◆ injuries inconsistent with what the child could do

- ◆ unusually shaped bruises or burns

- ◆ the child's apparent fear of the parent or caregiver

If you suspect child abuse, do not accuse anyone. Insist that the child receive medical help for their injuries. This will help ensure a full medical assessment. If you don't think the child will be taken to a doctor, call an ambulance and the police to the scene. This will help ensure a doctor sees the child.

If medical care for the child is refused and calling for an ambulance and/or the police is not possible, call a child welfare agency (often the Children's Aid Society) and report your suspicions. When you make such a call, giving your name is not required.

Help at an emergency scene

As a first aider, the first thing you do when you arrive at an emergency is take charge of the situation. You stay in charge until you hand control of the scene over to more qualified people. While in charge, many other people may offer to help.

Other first aiders - If another first aider arrives on the scene, they should tell you they are trained in first aid and ask if they can help. If someone arrives on scene and jumps right in, tell the person you are in charge, and ask if they want to help you.

If you feel another first aider at the scene is more qualified to handle the situation, ask that person to take control. On the other hand, the most qualified person does not need to be in control. The "first", first aider on the scene takes charge and stays in charge until they decide to hand over control.

Bystanders - Emergency scenes attract attention. There may be many people standing around. To give the casualty the safest care possible, only the people really needed should be at the scene. These include relatives and close friends of the casualty and any bystanders you ask to stay on the scene to help you. Everyone else should be asked to leave. If needed, have a bystander control the crowd.

Authorities (police, hydro) - Ambulance personnel, police officers and firefighters are known as first responders. It is their job to respond to an emergency. They are highly trained and will take charge of the scene as soon as they arrive. You can expect them to ask direct questions about the scene, the casualty and your involvement.

Other authorities may be called to the scene. For example, if there are downed power lines, electrical utility personnel will be called. In these situations, the other authorities have a defined role that is not necessarily to give care to any casualties.

Ten ways a bystander can help

. . . .

If you do not want to touch a casualty because of the risk of infection - is there anything you can do? Yes, there is plenty of first aid you can give. For example, you can:

1. Make the area safe
2. Find all the casualties
3. Find a first aid kit
4. Control the crowd
5. Call for medical help
6. Help give first aid, under your direction.
7. Gather and protect the casualty's belongings
8. Take notes
9. Reassure the casualty's relatives
10. Meet the ambulance and direct emergency person nel to the scene.

Off-duty doctors, nurses and other health professionals - Health professionals are a valuable source of help at an emergency scene. If someone identifies herself as a health professional and asks whether she can help, tell her you are a first aider and that you are in charge of the situation. If the health professional has training and experience in managing the type of illness or injury present, ask for her opinion and advice.

Always speak quietly so as not to alarm the casualty.

Medical help

Medical help is given by a medical doctor or given under the supervision of a medical doctor. Ambulance personnel give medical help because they work under the supervision of medical doctors. Medical help is given in hospitals but it can also be given at the emergency scene or on the way to a medical facility.

Sometimes the need for medical help is urgent - calling for medical help right away is necessary to save the casualty's life.

The Golden Hour refers to the first hour after the casualty has been injured. This time is "golden" because if the casualty with severe life-threatening injuries gets to a hospital within this hour, their chance of survival is "pretty good". After one hour, their chance for survival drops very quickly.

How to get medical help

Medical help is organized under a community's Emergency Medical Services (EMS) system. The EMS system is made up of many components including ambulance services, hospital emergency departments, doctors, ambulance personnel and fire fighters. As a first aider, you are also an important part of the community EMS system. It is your role to recognize an emergency, give first aid and call for help.

To be an effective first aider, you have to know how to get medical help quickly. Know the EMS telephone number for your community (often 911). If you are outside of your community, the EMS phone number(s) is listed in the first few pages of the telephone book. When you call, follow the dispatcher's instructions. Don't hang up until you are told to, or the dispatcher hangs up first.

Sending a bystander for medical help

If there is a bystander at the scene, it's best to send them to call for medical help. This allows you to stay at the scene and give first aid.

Tell the bystander:

◆ to call an ambulance - give them the phone number

◆ what's wrong with the casualty - give the worst possible situation to make sure the casualty gets the urgent care they may need

◆ where you are

◆ to report back to you - this way you know the call for medical help has been made

If possible, always send someone out to meet the ambulance. Leading the ambulance personnel to the emergency scene saves a lot of time.

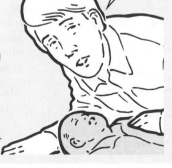

Call an ambulance. Dial 911 and tell them an infant is unresponsive. The address is 321 Oak Street. Hang up when they tell you to and then come back here.

Deciding to leave an unresponsive adult casualty to call medical help

Answer the questions below to help you decide whether you should leave the casualty to get medical help if you are alone.

start here

Is medical help nearby? (Meaning, can you get to a phone, call, and return within 3 minutes?)

NO

Stay with the casualty and give life-saving first aid. Once the casualty's life is out of immediate danger, decide whether to go—this is a judgement call, see opposite page.

YES

Can you carry the casualty while going to the phone?

NO

If the casualty is unresponsive , go for medical help. If you will be out of sight of the casualty, turn them into the recovery position before leaving.

YES

Go to call medical help, carrying the casualty with you.

If you are alone with a child or infant who is not breathing; perform 2 minutes of CPR before leaving to call for help

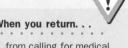

When you return. . .

. . .from calling for medical help, start first aid with the primary survey*—assessing and giving first aid for the ABCs*.

How ESM changes when a head or spinal injury is suspected

When there could be a head or spinal injury, protect the head and neck from any movement. Head or neck movement could result in life-long disability or death. Adjust your first aid to this situation as shown below.

1

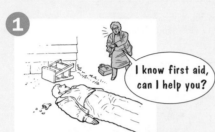

I know first aid, can I help you?

As soon as you see there might be a head or spinal injury, tell the casualty not to move.

2

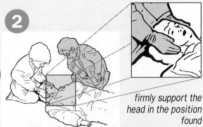

firmly support the head in the position found

Once you have consent to help the casualty, steady and support the head and neck. Then, assess responsiveness.

3

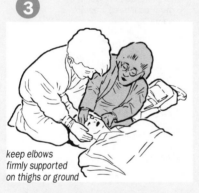

keep elbows firmly supported on thighs or ground

If there is a bystander to help, show them how to support the head and neck so you can continue your assessment.

4

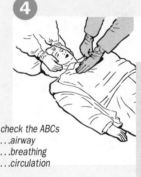

*check the ABCs
...airway
...breathing
...circulation*

If the casualty is unresponsive, check breathing in the position found before opening the airway. If there is no breathing, open the airway using a jaw thrust without head tilt and check breathing again.

Continue your assessment —check the ABCs.

5

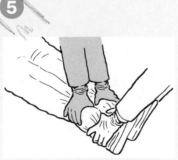

If a second bystander is available, show them how to steady and support the feet to prevent movement.

6

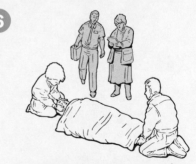

Keep the head and neck supported (and the feet if possible) while giving further first aid until handover to medical help, or until the casualty is completely immobilized on a long spine board.

Emergency scene management

Imagine a busy restaurant at lunchtime—people eating quickly and servers hurrying to get them on their way as fast as possible. Suddenly there is a commotion, and you see a woman lying on the ground... what happens now?

Emergency scenes like this usually begin with a lot of confusion as people realize there is an emergency unfolding in front of them—no one knows what to do first, who should be in charge or how they can help. In this situation, the first aider needs to follow a sequence of actions that ensure safe and appropriate first aid is given and everyone's safety is protected. St. John Ambulance first aiders use **emergency scene management** (called ESM for short) to do this.

ESM has four steps:

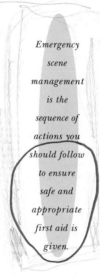

Emergency scene management is the sequence of actions you should follow to ensure safe and appropriate first aid is given.

- *scene survey*—here you take control of the scene and find out what happened before helping any casualties

- *primary survey*—here you assess each casualty for life-threatening injuries or illnesses and give life-saving first aid

- *secondary survey*—during this step the first aider performs a more thorough check for injuries and illnesses that were not revealed in the primary survey, but would benefit from first aid

- *ongoing casualty care*—here you stay with the casualty until medical help arrives and takes over

These steps are always done in the order above, though sometimes you don't do the secondary survey.

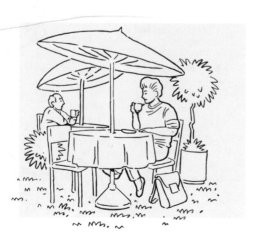

Emergency scene management

Emergency scene management (ESM) is the sequence of actions you should take at the scene of an emergency to ensure that safe and appropriate first aid is given. Following the steps will help you make rapid and accurate decisions to give the best possible care to the casualty.

ESM has many steps and can be quite complicated, but the initial scene survey, primary survey and the start of life-saving first aid usually happens very quickly—within one or two minutes.

Scene survey

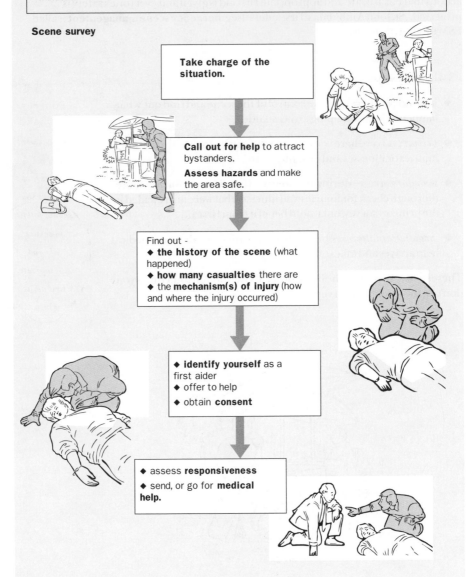

Take charge of the situation.

Call out for help to attract bystanders.

Assess hazards and make the area safe.

Find out -

◆ **the history of the scene** (what happened)

◆ **how many casualties** there are

◆ the **mechanism(s) of injury** (how and where the injury occurred)

◆ **identify yourself** as a first aider

◆ offer to help

◆ obtain **consent**

◆ assess **responsiveness**

◆ send, or go for **medical help.**

Primary survey

The primary survey is the first step in assessing the casualty for life-threatening conditions and giving life-saving first aid.

In the primary survey, you check for the **priorities of first aid**:

- ◆ Airway - to ensure a clear airway
- ◆ Breathing - to ensure effective breathing
- ◆ Circulation - to ensure effective circulation

Even if there is more than one casualty, perform a primary survey on each casualty. Give life-saving first aid only.

The sequential steps of the primary survey should be performed with the casualty in the **position found** unless it is impossssible to do so. Give first aid for life-threatening conditions as you find them while checking the ABCs.

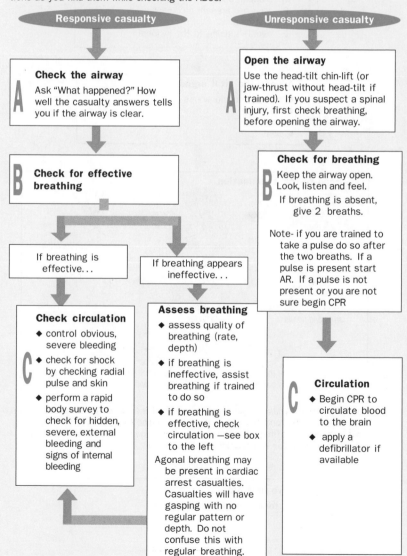

Responsive casualty

Check the airway

Ask "What happened?" How well the casualty answers tells you if the airway is clear.

Check for effective breathing

If breathing is effective...

If breathing appears ineffective...

Check circulation

- ◆ control obvious, severe bleeding
- ◆ check for shock by checking radial pulse and skin
- ◆ perform a rapid body survey to check for hidden, severe, external bleeding and signs of internal bleeding

Assess breathing

- ◆ assess quality of breathing (rate, depth)
- ◆ if breathing is ineffective, assist breathing if trained to do so
- ◆ if breathing is effective, check circulation —see box to the left

Agonal breathing may be present in cardiac arrest casualties. Casualties will have gasping with no regular pattern or depth. Do not confuse this with regular breathing.

Unresponsive casualty

Open the airway

Use the head-tilt chin-lift (or jaw-thrust without head-tilt if trained). If you suspect a spinal injury, first check breathing, before opening the airway.

Check for breathing

Keep the airway open. Look, listen and feel.
If breathing is absent, give 2 breaths.

Note- if you are trained to take a pulse do so after the two breaths. If a pulse is present start AR. If a pulse is not present or you are not sure begin CPR

Circulation

- ◆ Begin CPR to circulate blood to the brain
- ◆ apply a defibrillator if available

Secondary survey

The secondary survey is a step-by-step way of gathering information to form a complete picture of the condition of the casualty. At this stage, you are looking for injuries and illnesses that were not revealed in the primary survey, but could benefit from first aid.

After giving first aid for life-threatening injuries, do a secondary survey if medical help is delayed more than 20 minutes, if you have to transport the casualty or the casualty has more than one injury. This step may be omitted if first aid for life-threatening conditions has been given and medical help is close by.

History of the casualty

1

S   symptoms
A   allergies
M   medications
P   past and present medical history
L   last meal
E   events leading to the incident

Assess the vital signs

2

◆ level of consciousness
◆ breathing
◆ pulse
◆ skin

Head-to-toe examination

3

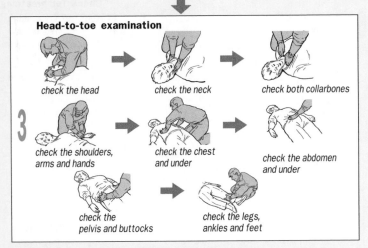

check the head   check the neck   check both collarbones

check the shoulders,   check the chest   check the abdomen
arms and hands   and under   and under

check the   check the legs,
pelvis and buttocks   ankles and feet

Do not examine for unlikely injuries. For example, if the casualty cut their hand with a knife while preparing food, there is no need to examine for injuries to the legs. Consider the history of the situation and the signs and symptoms to decide how much of the head-to-toe examination you need to do.

Give first aid. . .

4

. . . for injuries or illnesses found

Ongoing Casualty Care

Once the first aid for non-life threatening injuries and illnesses has been given, one of three things happens:

◆ you hand over control of the scene to the casualty, or someone else, and end your involvement in the emergency
◆ you stay in control of the scene and wait for medical help to arrive and take over
◆ you stay in control of the scene and transport the casualty to medical help.

When you stay in control of the scene, you continue to give first aid. You must maintain the casualty in the best possible condition until hand over to medical help.

Instruct a bystander to maintain manual support of the head and neck, if head/spinal injuries are suspected.

Continue to steady and support any injuries manually, if needed.

1 **Give first aid for shock**
◆ reassure the casualty
◆ loosen tight clothing
◆ place the casualty in the best position for the condition
◆ cover the casualty to preserve body heat

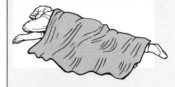

2 **Monitor the casualty's condition**
◆ check the ABCs often
◆ give nothing by mouth

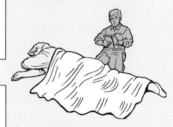

3 **Record the events of the situation**
◆ protect the casualty's belongings

4 **Report on what happened**
◆ tell whoever takes over what happened, what kind of injuries are involved and what first aid has been given

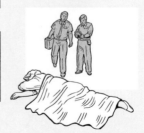

> ⚠ Do not leave the casualty until you hand control of the scene over to someone else.

How to put a casualty into the recovery position—method 1

The recovery position keeps an unconscious person's airway open. Always put a semi-conscious or unconscious person into the recovery position if you cannot constantly monitor the person's breathing. The method below is the preferred one.

1

place the near arm straight out

place the far arm with the back of the hand over the near cheek

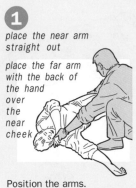

Position the arms.

2

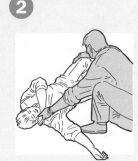

Bend and grab the far knee.

3

protect the casualty's head during the roll

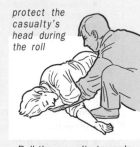

Roll the casualty towards you by pulling the far knee towards you and to the ground.

4

adjust the hand under the head so the neck is extended

5

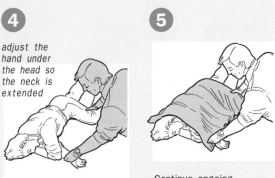

Continue ongoing casualty care.

How to put a casualty into the recovery position—method 2

Use this method only if the casualty is much larger than you and too heavy to roll using method 1.

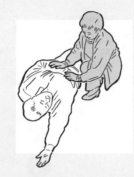

Position the arm closest to you.

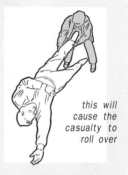

Position the arm furthest from you.

this will cause the casualty to roll over

Pick up the far lower leg and walk it around and over the casualty's near leg.

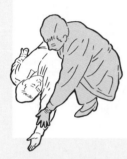

Position this leg with the knee bent.

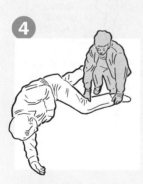

Position the arms to keep the neck extended.

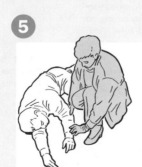

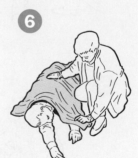

Continue ongoing casualty care.

How to put a casualty into the Haines position

Use the HAINES (high arm in endangered spine) if you suspect a spinal injury. Only put the casualty in this position to protect the airway (e.g you must leave the casualty to activate EMS). This method helps reduce bending and twisting of the spine when rolling the casualty over.

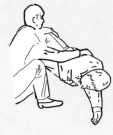

Position the arm closest to you with the arm above the casualty's head.

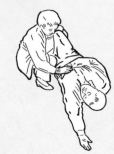

Position the arm furthest from you on the casualty's chest and bend the far knee

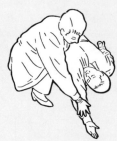

Reach behind the casualty's shoulder and roll the casualty towards you by pulling on the far knee

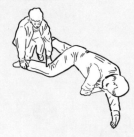

Place the far arm at 90 degrees to the casualty with the palm face down. Place padding behind casualty to prevent them from rolling back into a face up position.

Adjust the position of the arms and leg so the casualty is in a stable position.

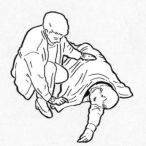

Give on-going care

Sample first aid report form

First Aid Report

Date _____

Location _____

First aider

Name _____

Address _____

City _____

Province _____ Postal code _____

Telephone number _____

Casualty

Name _____

Address _____

City _____

Province _____ Postal code _____

Telephone number _____

☐ Male ☐ Female Age (approx.) _____

Scene survey

Type of incident _____

Number of casualties _____
(use a separate form for each casualty)

Casualty responsiveness
☐ responsive ☐ unresponsive

Primary survey

Airway
☐ clear
☐ partly blocked
☐ completely blocked

Breathing
☐ yes.... ☐ effective ☐ ineffective
☐ no

Circulation
Pulse ☐ yes ☐ no
Severe bleeding ☐ yes ☐ no
Shock ☐ yes ☐ no

Secondary survey

History
Symptoms _____
_____
Allergies _____
Medications _____
Past medical history _____
Last meal _____
Events leading to incident _____
_____

Vital signs
Time taken _____ _____ _____
Level of consc. _____ _____ _____
Breathing rate _____ _____ _____
Breathing rhythm _____ _____ _____
Breathing depth _____ _____ _____
Pulse rate _____ _____ _____
Pulse rhythm _____ _____ _____
Pulse strength _____ _____ _____
Skin cond./temp. _____ _____ _____

Head-to-toe examination
Head _____
Neck _____
Collarbones _____
Shoulders arms/hands _____
Chest and under _____
Abdomen and under _____
Pelvis and buttocks _____
Legs/feet _____

First aid given

_____
_____
_____
_____
_____

Hand over to medical help

_____
_____
_____
_____
_____
_____

Emergency Scene Management - Activity

1. ___First AID___ is emergency help given to an injured or suddenly ill person using readily available materials.

2. The objectives of first aid are to:

   a) _____.

   b) _____.

   c) _____.

3. _____ is given by a medical doctor or given under the supervision of a medical doctor.

Legal and Safety Issues

4. The principles of the Good Samaritan include:

   a) _____.

   b) _____.

   c) _____.

   d) _____.

5. The universal precautions that apply to first aiders are:

   a) _____.

   b) _____.

   c) _____.

6. When giving first aid as part of your job, you **have / don't have** a legal duty to respond to an emergency situation at your workplace. *(Circle your choice.)*

7. In Canada (except Quebec) and most of the United States, A first aider **has / doesn't have** a legal duty to help a person in need. *(Circle your choice.)*

8. In a violent or potentially violent situation, your first priority as a first aider is to

   _____.

Emergency Scene Management - Activity

Emergency Scene Management

9. _____ is the sequence of actions you should take at the scene of an emergency to ensure that safe and appropriate first aid is given.

10. The steps of Emergency Scene Management (ESM) are:

    a) *Survey*

    b) *Primary Survey*

    c) *Secondary Survey*

    d) *On going care*

11. In the primary survey, you check for the **priorities of first aid**:

    a) _____ .

    b) _____ .

    c) _____ .

12. Wherever possible the casualty should be in the _____
    (position of the casualty) while you complete the primary survey.

13. The secondary survey should be done if:

    a) _____ .

    b) _____ .

    c) _____ .

14. The four steps of the secondary survey are:

    a) _____ .

    b) _____ .

    c) _____ .

    d) _____ .

15. The four steps of ongoing casualty care are:

    a) _____ .

    b) _____ .

    c) _____ .

    d) _____ .

Emergency Scene Management - Activity

16. You come across a young woman lying on the ground outside her home. Describe the steps you would take beginning with your approach and continuing until you handover control to medical help.

The first step in the scene survey is to _____ of the situation.

In assessing the _____ of the incident, a bystander tells you the woman fell from a step ladder.

When there could be a head or spinal injury, you should protect the _____ and _____ from any movement.

Ask a bystander to call for _____ .

PRIMARY SURVEY

You check the ABCs and determine the casualty is breathing and has adequate circulation.

SECONDARY SURVEY

Medical help is expected right away. You **should / should not** proceed with a secondary survey at this point. *(Circle your choice.)*

ONGOING CARE

Following first aid, you should monitor the casualty's condition. When medical help arrives you should provide information on:

a) _____ .

b) _____ .

c) _____ .

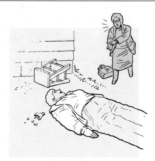

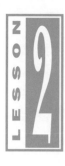

LESSON 2

Objectives

◆ Recognize shock

◆ Provide first aid for shock

◆ Recognize unconsciousness

◆ Provide first aid for unconsciousness

◆ Recognize fainting

◆ Provide first aid for fainting

Shock

Any injury or illness can be accompanied by shock. Shock is a circulation problem where the body's tissues don't get enough blood. This is medical shock—don't confuse it with an electric shock or "being shocked" as in scared or surprised. Medical shock is life threatening because the brain and other organs cannot function properly. If shock gets bad enough, it leads to unconsciousness and even death. Because there is often shock in an emergency situation, and because it can progress very quickly, always check for shock and assess whether it is getting bad enough to be a medical emergency by itself. Like safety, shock is one of those things you always have to be thinking about.

Common causes of severe shock	
Cause of shock	**How it causes a circulation problem**
severe bleeding - internal or external (includes major fractures)	not enough blood to fill blood vessels
severe burns	loss of blood plasma (fluid) into tissues—not enough blood to fill blood vessels
crush injuries	loss of blood and blood plasma into tissues—not enough blood to fill blood vessels
heart attack	heart is not strong enough to pump blood properly
spinal cord or nerve injuries	brain can't control the size of the blood vessels and the blood can't get to the tissues properly
severe allergic reactions	many things can be affected—breathing, heart function, etc.

The table above gives some causes of shock. Severe shock can also result from medical emergencies such as diabetes, epilepsy, infection, poisoning or a drug overdose. Pain, anxiety and fear don't cause shock, but they can help make it worse, or make it progress faster. This is why reassuring a casualty and making them comfortable is so important.

Signs and symptoms of shock

Signs

pale skin at first,
turns bluish-grey

bluish-purple lips,
tongue, earlobes,
fingernails

cold and clammy
skin

breathing shallow &
irregular, fast or
gasping for air

changes in level of
consciousness

weak, rapid pulse—
radial pulse may be
absent

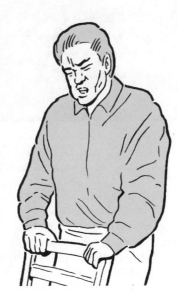

Symptoms

restless

anxious

disoriented

confused

afraid

dizzy

thirsty, may be
very thirsty

Minimizing shock

The following actions will minimize shock:

1 Give first aid for the injury or illness that caused the shock.

2 Reassure the casualty often.

3 Minimize pain by handling the casualty gently.

4 Loosen tight clothing at the neck, chest and waist.

5 Keep the casualty warm, but do not overheat—use jackets, coats, or blankets if you have them.

6 Moisten the lips if the casualty complains of thirst—don't give anything to eat or drink. If medical help is delayed many hours, give water or clear fluids to drink—make a note of what was given and when.

7 Place the casualty in the best position for their condition—see the positions on the next page.

8 Continue ongoing casualty care until handover.

The above first aid for shock also prevents shock from getting worse. Whenever possible, add these steps to any first aid you give—this will minimize shock.

Positioning a casualty in shock

Putting the casualty in the right position can slow the progress of shock and make the casualty more comfortable. The position you use depends on the casualty's condition. The casualty should be as comfortable as possible in the position you use.

No suspected head/spinal injury; fully conscious

Place the casualty on their back with feet and legs raised—this position is often called the **shock position**. Once the casualty is positioned, cover them to preserve body heat, but do not overheat.

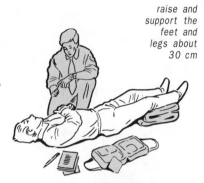

raise and support the feet and legs about 30 cm

No suspected head/spinal injury; less than fully conscious

Place the casualty in the recovery position—see pages 1-16 to 1-18. When there is a decreased level of consciousness, airway and breathing are the priority—the recovery position ensures an open airway.

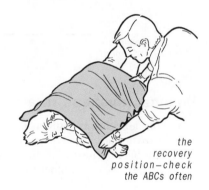

Suspected head/spinal injury

If there might be a head or spinal injury, steady and support the casualty in the position found and monitor the ABCs closely. This protects the head and spine from further injury.

the recovery position—check the ABCs often

As injuries permit

A casualty's injuries may not permit you to put them into the best position. For instance, raising the legs of a person with a fractured pelvis can cause more pain and aggravate the injury. Keep this person lying flat on their back. If trained, put them on a stretcher, or a backboard, and raise the foot of the stretcher. Always think of the casualty's comfort when choosing a position.

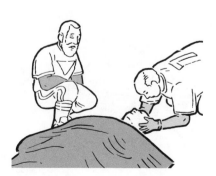

Level of consciousness (LOC)

Consciousness means how aware a person is of them self and their surroundings. There is a full range of levels of consciousness, from completely conscious to completely unconscious. Many injuries and illnesses can cause changes in a casualty's level of consciousness. Some examples are:

- a breathing emergency
- a heart attack
- a head injury
- poisoning
- shock
- alcohol or drug abuse
- a medical condition (epilepsy, diabetes, etc.)

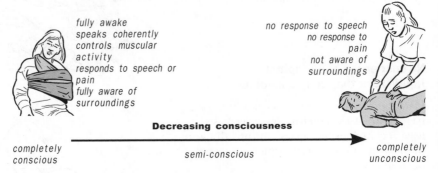

fully awake
speaks coherently
controls muscular activity
responds to speech or pain
fully aware of surroundings

no response to speech
no response to pain
not aware of surroundings

Decreasing consciousness

completely
conscious

semi-conscious

completely
unconscious

Unconsciousness is a medical emergency

Semi-consciousness and unconsciousness are medical emergencies because the tongue may fall to the back of the throat and block the airway. Also, saliva and other fluids can pool at the back of the throat. Since an unconscious person loses the reflex to cough up fluids in the throat, they block the airway and choke the person.

A progressive loss of consciousness means the casualty's condition is getting worse. Always monitor a casualty's level of consciousness and note any changes.

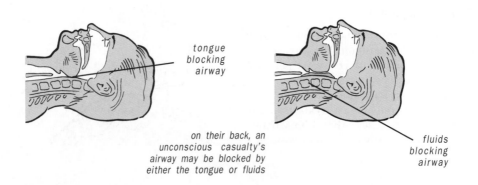

tongue
blocking
airway

on their back, an
unconscious casualty's
airway may be blocked by
either the tongue or fluids

fluids
blocking
airway

Assessing level of consciousness

A first aider uses the **Modified Glasgow Coma Scale** to assess and describe levels of consciousness. The scale is based on the casualty's ability:

- to open the eyes—this is the **eye opening response**
- to speak—this is the **verbal response**
- to move muscles—this is the **motor response**

Use the information below to determine whether the casualty is conscious, semi-conscious or unconscious.

	When a person is **conscious. . .**	When a person is **semi-conscious. . .**	When the person is **unconscious. . .**
Eye opening response	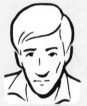 . . . eyes open spontaneously	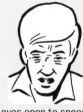 . . . eyes open to speech or pain	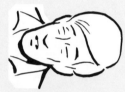 . . . eyes don't open
Verbal response	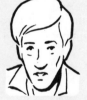 . . . is oriented and alert	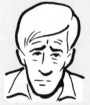 . . . is confused, doesn't make sense	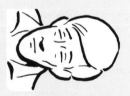 . . . is not aware of his surroundings
Motor response	. . . obeys commands	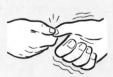 . . . reacts to pain but does not obey commands	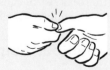 . . . doesn't react to pain

First aid for semi-consciousness and unconsciousness

1   Start ESM—do a scene survey. Have a bystander call for medical help as soon as unresponsiveness is recognized. See page 1-9 for what to do if you are alone.

2   Do a primary survey and give life-saving first aid.

3   Do a secondary survey if necessary and give first aid.

4   Turn the casualty into the recovery position, if injuries permit. If injuries make it better for the casualty to be face up, monitor breathing continuously.

5   Loosen tight clothing at the neck, chest and waist, and continue ongoing casualty care until hand over. Record any changes in level of consciousness and when they happen.

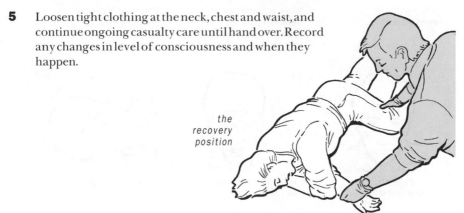

the recovery position

Always ensure an open airway. If the casualty's injuries permit, put them into the recovery position. Otherwise, closely monitor breathing. Sometimes you cannot monitor the casualty's breathing.

For instance, if:

◆ you have to leave to get medical help

◆ you have to give first aid to other casualties

Here, turn the casualty into the recovery position, being as careful as you can if there are any injuries.

Although there is a risk of causing more injury, keeping the airway open is more important and must be your first concern.

Urgent medical help required

Decreased consciousness is always an urgent situation. The person can quickly become unconscious, and this is a medical emergency. When you recognize decreased consciousness, get medical help as fast as possible.

Fainting

Fainting is a loss of consciousness that lasts a very short time—no more than a few minutes. It is caused by a temporary shortage of oxygenated blood to the brain. Some common reasons people faint are:

- fear or anxiety
- severe pain, injury or illness
- underlying medical problem
- long periods of standing or sitting

- lack of fresh air
- the sight of blood
- fatigue or hunger

A person losing consciousness is always a serious medical emergency. Do not assume a person has "just fainted" until there is a quick, full recovery and the reason for the fainting is known. If you think there might be a serious reason a person feels faint, or has fainted, get medical help.

Feels faint or "impending faint"

Sometimes when a person is about to faint, there are warning signs. The person:

- is pale
- is sweating
- feels sick, nauseous, dizzy and unsteady

When a person is about to faint, act quickly.

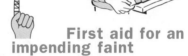

First aid for an impending faint

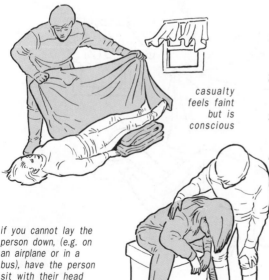

casualty feels faint but is conscious

if you cannot lay the person down, (e.g. on an airplane or in a bus), have the person sit with their head lower than their shoulders

1 Lay the casualty down with the feet raised about 30 cm (12 in).

2 Ensure a supply of fresh air— open windows or doors.

3 Loosen tight clothing at the neck, chest and waist.

4 Stay with the casualty until fully recovered.

First aid for fainting

A person who has fainted is unconscious. The first aid for fainting is the same as the first aid for unconsciousness.

1 Start ESM—do a scene survey. Have a bystander call for medical help as soon as unresponsiveness is recognized. See page 1-9 for what to do if you are alone.

2 Check the ABCs—make sure the casualty's airway is clear, that they are breathing effectively, and check for shock.

3 Do a secondary survey if necessary and give first aid.

4 Turn the casualty into the recovery position, if injuries permit (see pages 1-16 to 1-18).

5 Ensure a supply of fresh air and loosen tight clothing at the neck, chest and waist. Continue ongoing casualty care until hand over.

6 Make the casualty comfortable as consciousness returns and keep them lying down for 10 to 15 minutes.

Recovery from a faint should be quick and complete. If this is not the case, stay with the casualty until medical help takes over.

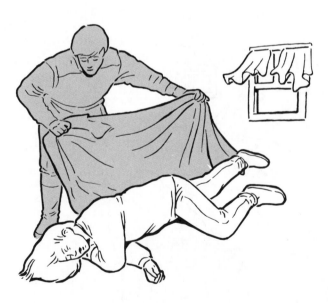

casualty is unconscious

Shock, Unconsciousness and Fainting - Activity

• •

• • • • • • • • • •   **Shock**   • • • • • • • • • •

1. _____ is a circulation problem where the body tissues don't get enough blood. Shock can lead to _____ or _____.

2. Causes of shock include:

    a) _____   b) _____

    c) _____   d) _____.

3. Signs and symptoms of shock include:

    a) _____   b) _____

    c) _____   d) _____.

4. The position you chose to reduce shock depends on _____.

5. Actions you should take to reduce shock in the casualty include:

    a) _____

    b) _____

    c) _____

    d) _____

    e) _____

    f) _____

    g) _____

    h) _____.

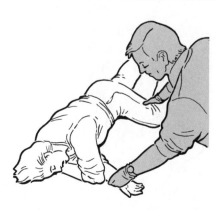

Shock, Unconsciousness and Fainting - Activity - (cont.)

• •

· · · · · · · · · **Unconsciousness** · · · · · · · ·

6. **Unconsciousness** may be a _____ emergency. It is important to get _____ as fast as possible.

7. Level of consciousness can be assessed according to the casualty's abilities in three areas:

   a) _____ .

   b) _____ .

   c) _____ .

8. If injuries permit, the unconscious casualty should be placed in the _____ position.

· · · · · · · · · · **Fainting** · · · · · · · · · ·

9. **Fainting** is a _____ that lasts a very short time.

10. You should recognize that the casualty may faint if they are _____, are _____ and/or feels _____ .

11. If the person feels faint they should be positioned _____ with the feet _____ .

12. If the casualty faints, give first aid as for _____ .

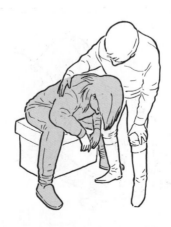

2-10

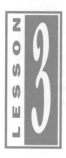

Objectives

◆ Take measures to prevent choking

◆ Recognize choking

◆ Provide first aid for an adult choking casualty

◆ Provide ongoing casualty care and hand over for a casualty whose airway has been cleared

Introduction

A person chokes when the airway is partly or completely blocked and airflow to the lungs is reduced or cut off. The choking casualty either has trouble breathing or cannot breathe at all. A choking casualty may die if first aid for choking is not given right away.

Air exchange – good, poor or none

A person's airway can be either partly or completely blocked. With a partially blocked airway, there is either **good air exchange** or **poor air exchange**. With good air exchange, the obstruction is **mild** and person can still cough forcefully, breathe and speak. With poor air exchange, the obstruction is **severe** and the person cannot cough forcefully, has trouble breathing, or cannot speak. With a completely blocked airway, there is no air exchange—coughing, breathing and speaking are impossible.

airway is open and clear

partly blocked airway

partial blockage

completely blocked airway

foreign object

Causes of choking

Foreign objects	Unconscious casualty	Injury or illness
◆ in infants and children—food, toys, buttons, coins, etc.	◆ tongue falls to the back of the throat when lying on back	◆ injury to the throat area causes swelling of the airway

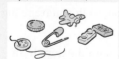

◆ in adults—gulping drinks with food in your mouth

◆ in elderly people—food, pills

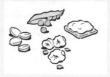

◆ saliva, blood or vomit pools in the throat

◆ illness causes swelling, e.g. allergic reaction, asthma, epiglottitis, croup

swollen airway

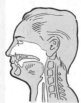

What happens when a person chokes

Choking is a life-threatening emergency. When the air supply to the lungs is cut off, the person's face immediately becomes reddish. Shortly after, as the oxygen in the body is used up, the face becomes grey and the lips and ear lobes become bluish. This change in colour is called **cyanosis**. Soon, the person becomes unconscious and eventually the heart stops beating.

Signs of choking

The most obvious sign of choking is grabbing the throat. The other signs are given in the illustration below. Notice how they are different with mild or severe obstructions.

You need to know how to recognize whether a choking person has a mild or severe obstruction because the first aid is different for each.

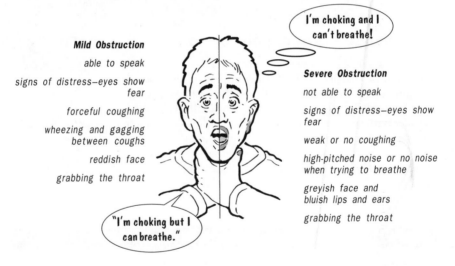

Mild Obstruction

able to speak

signs of distress—eyes show fear

forceful coughing

wheezing and gagging between coughs

reddish face

grabbing the throat

"I'm choking but I can breathe."

I'm choking and I can't breathe!

Severe Obstruction

not able to speak

signs of distress—eyes show fear

weak or no coughing

high-pitched noise or no noise when trying to breathe

greyish face and bluish lips and ears

grabbing the throat

There are two choking situations you may have to deal with:

◆ a conscious choking person who may become unconscious while you are giving first aid

◆ an unconscious person who, you discover through your first aid actions, has a blocked airway

The first aid you give depends on the casualty's age. In first aid for choking, an adult is over the age of eight, a child is between one and eight years of age, and an infant is under one year old. These ages are guidelines only; the casualty's size must be also considered. There are variations in the techniques for a casualty who is pregnant or much larger than the rescuer or in a wheelchair.

Choking adult – conscious who may become unconscious

1 Begin ESM—do a scene survey.

2 If the casualty can cough forcefully, speak or breathe, don't touch them. Tell them to try to cough up the object. If a mild obstruction lasts for a few minutes, get medical help.

> If choking is caused by swelling of the airway from an infection, injury or allergic reaction, abdominal thrusts won't work—get medical help quickly.

If you think there might be a severe obstruction, check by asking, "Are you choking?" If the casualty cannot cough forcefully, speak or breathe, use abdominal thrusts to try to remove the blockage—go to step 3.

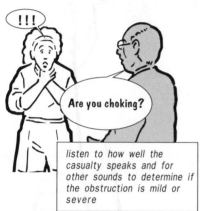

listen to how well the casualty speaks and for other sounds to determine if the obstruction is mild or severe

3 Stand behind the casualty ready to support them if they become unconscious. Find the correct hand position and give abdominal thrusts to try to remove the airway blockage.

Give each abdominal thrust with the intention of removing the object. Use only your fist—make sure you don't press against the ribs with your forearms.

4 Keep giving abdominal thrusts until either the object is removed or the casualty becomes unconscious. If the airway is cleared, give ongoing casualty care for choking.

If the casualty becomes unconscious, don't panic. Continue first aid with step 5 on the next page.

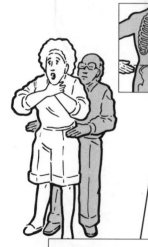

find the top of the hip bones

place a foot between the casualty's feet for a solid position

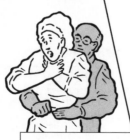

place your fist midline, just above the other hand

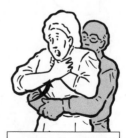

hold the fist with the other hand and press inward/upward with a sudden, forceful thrust—this is an abdominal thrust

5 As the casualty collapses, lower them to the ground. Send someone to call for medical help and get an AED if available.

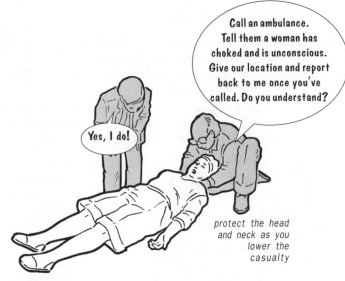

Call an ambulance. Tell them a woman has choked and is unconscious. Give our location and report back to me once you've called. Do you understand?

Yes, I do!

protect the head and neck as you lower the casualty

6 Open the mouth and look for any foreign matter. If you see something, remove it. Open the airway and assess for normal breathing for no more than ten seconds.

hold the mouth open

look in the mouth for a foreign object

remove any foreign matter — pull it up against the near cheek— be careful, the object may be sharp or slippery

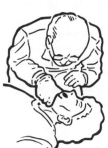

open the airway by tilting the head back and lifting the jaw

with the ear just above the mouth, look, listen and feel for signs of breathing

7 Try to breathe into the casualty's mouth.

push back on the forehead and lift the jaw

seal your mouth around the casualty's mouth

pinch the nostrils

blow in—watch for the chest to rise

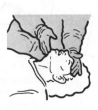

if the chest doesn't rise, reposition the head, check the seals at the nose and mouth and try again.

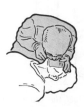

if the chest doesn't rise on your second try, conclude the airway is blocked—try to clear the airway—go to step 8

8   Begin chest compressions. Give 30 compressions.

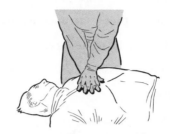

kneel so your hands can be
placed mid-chest

place 2 hands in the centre
of the upper chest and give
30 compressions

- -

9   Repeat looking in the mouth, attempting to ventilate and giving chest
compressions

look in the mouth

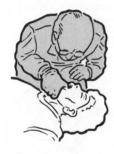

tilt the head and try to
ventilate twice

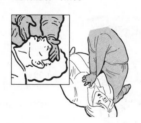

give chest
compressions

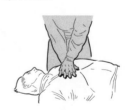

- -

10 If you remove the blockage or if the chest rises when
you ventilate, give two breaths. If there is no response (e.g casualty starts to breathe) continue with
the normal CPR sequence. If the casualty begins to
respond give the ongoing casualty care described on
page 3-10.

If an AED is available
apply the device as
soon as possible and
follow the voice
prompts from the
machine. The CPR
sequence remains the
same except that the
first aider checks the
mouth each time
before attempting to
give a breath

Choking adult – found unconscious

You arrive at a scene. . .there is an unconscious person lying on the floor. . .

1 Begin ESM—start the scene survey.

2 Assess responsiveness.

Are you O.K.?

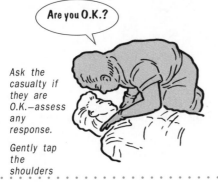

Ask the casualty if they are O.K.–assess any response.

Gently tap the shoulders

3 Send or go for medical help and an AED if available. See page 1-9 for what to do if you are alone.

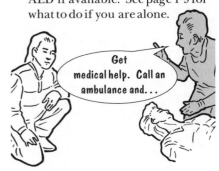

Get medical help. Call an ambulance and. . .

4 If necessary, turn the casualty face up. Open the airway.

push backward on the forehead and lift the jaw

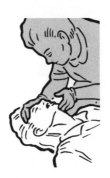

5 Check for normal breathing for up to 10 seconds.

keep the head tilted

with your ear close to the casualty's mouth and nose, check for breathing

look. . . for chest movement

listen. . . for sounds of breathing

feel. . . for breath on your cheek

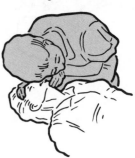

6 Try to breathe into the casualty's mouth.

push back on the forehead and lift the jaw

seal your mouth around the casualty's mouth

pinch the nostrils

blow in–watch for the chest to rise

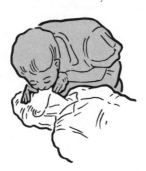

if the chest doesn't rise, reposition the head, check the seals at the nose and mouth and try again.

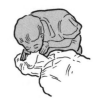

if the chest doesn't rise on your second try, conclude the airway is blocked–try to clear the airway–go to step 7

7 Begin chest compressions. Place hands in the correct position, and give 30 compressions.

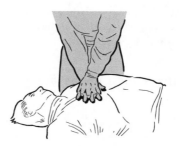

kneel so your hands can be placed mid-chest

place 2 hands in the centre of the upper chest and give 30 compressions

8 Open the mouth and look for the foreign object. If you see it, remove it. Attempt 2 ventilations. If air won't go in give 30 compressions.

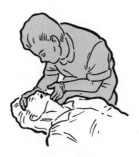

9 Repeat looking in the mouth, attempting to ventilate and giving chest compressions.

If you remove the blockage or if the chest rises when you ventilate, give two breaths. If there is no response (e.g casualty starts to breathe) continue with the normal CPR sequence. If the casualty begins to respond give the ongoing casualty care described on page 3-10.

If an AED is available apply the device as soon as possible and follow the voice prompts from the machine. The CPR sequence remains the same except that the first aider checks the mouth each time before attempting to give a breath

Choking adult – first aid for larger or pregnant choking casualties

If a choking casualty is much larger than the rescuer or if the casualty is in the late stages of pregnancy, abdominal thrusts may not be effective. Instead of abdominal thrusts, use chest thrusts as described below.

Chest thrusts for a conscious choking casualty

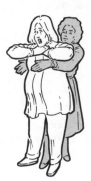

stand behind the casualty

wrap your arms around the chest

keep arms horizontal and snug up under the armpits

place your fist against the lower half of the breastbone, thumb-side in

hold the fist with your other hand

pull inward forcefully

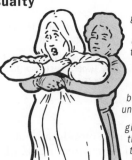

give chest thrusts until either the object is removed or the casualty becomes unconscious

give each thrust with the intention of removing the blockage

Chest compressions for an unconscious choking casualty

kneel so your hands can be placed mid-chest

place 2 hands in the centre of the upper chest and give 30 compressions

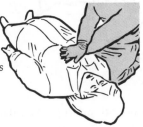

 ### Positioning a pregnant casualty

Whenever a pregnant casualty is positioned face up, place something like a jacket or a pillow, if you have one, under the right hip. This positions the baby off an important blood vessel in the mother.

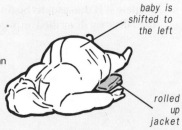

baby is shifted to the left

rolled up jacket

Choking adult – first aid for a casualty in a wheelchair

The way you do abdominal thrusts for someone in a wheelchair depends largely on the type of wheelchair. If you can reach around from behind the wheelchair, use abdominal thrusts as you would for any conscious casualty of the same age. If you cannot reach around the wheelchair, use the technique shown below.

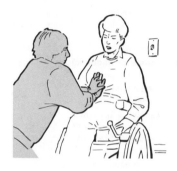

position the wheelchair against a wall

put the wheelchair brake on

put the heel of one hand, with the other on top, in the middle of the abdomen

give sudden, inward/upward thrusts until the object is removed or the casualty becomes unconscious

If the casualty becomes unconscious, take them out of the wheelchair.

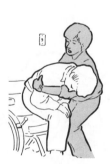

pull the casualty forward supporting them with your arm and leg

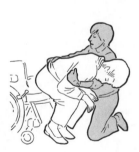

grip the casualty's clothing

lower yourself and the casualty to the ground using the strength in your legs and not your back as much as possible

If a doctor, physiotherapist or other health professional has shown you a different way of giving abominal thrusts to a person in your care, use the method that you prefer.

supporting the casualty, and protecting the head as much as possible, roll the casualty to the floor to a face-up position

when she is face up, give first aid for choking—go to step 6, page 3-6

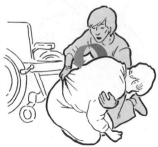

Ongoing casualty care for choking

Your job as a first aider is not over when the airway blockage is removed. When a choking casualty's airway has been cleared, they may be conscious, semi-conscious or unconscious. Continue giving first aid as described below.

If the casualty is conscious

- monitor breathing often. Breathing difficulties can develop following a choking incident
- stay with the casualty until normal breathing returns
- urge the casualty to see a medical doctor—abdominal thrusts can cause internal injuries

If the casualty is semi-conscious or unconscious

- call for medical help if not called already
- if the casualty is breathing, place them in the recovery position and give first aid for shock
- stay with the casualty until medical help takes over
- monitor ABCs

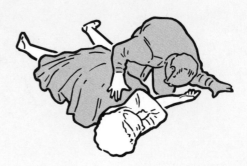

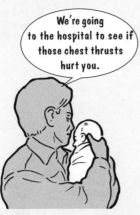

Choking adult – self-help

If you begin to choke on an object, what should you do?

1 Don't panic, though that's not easy. If there are people around, get their attention—grab your throat to show them you are choking—this is the universal sign of choking. **Do not isolate yourself from others when you are choking**.

2 If you can cough forcefully, try to cough up the object. Don't let anyone slap you on the back, this could drive the object further down your airway.

3 If you can't cough forcefully, breathe or speak, and there is no one else to give you abdominal thrusts, do it to yourself as shown below. Use either your hands or a piece of furniture, whatever gives the best effect.

If you are alone and choking, you must get help quickly—you will become unconscious within minutes.

Do whatever is necessary to get someone's attention. If all else fails, and you have 911 emergency service in your area, call 911.

In some areas, the 911 operator can see on her equipment the address of the phone the caller is using and will send help even though you cannot tell them what's wrong.

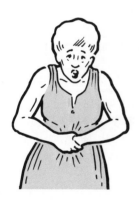

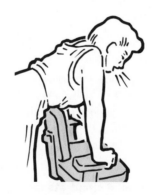

put a fist, thumb-side in, midline on your abdomen just above your hips

hold the fist with your other hand and pull inward/upward forcefully

give yourself abdominal thrusts until you can cough forcefully, breathe or speak

a second method is to use a solid object like the back of a chair, a table or the edge of a counter

position yourself so the object is just above your hips. Press forcefully to produce an abdominal thrust—keep giving yourself thrusts until you can cough forcefully, breathe or speak

If you are very large or in the late stages of pregnancy, give yourself chest thrusts instead. Place a fist, thumb-side down, in the middle of your chest. With your head turned to the side, fall against a wall hard enough to produce a chest thrust.

Choking - Activity

Conscious who may become unconscious

1. If the obstruction is mild, you **should / should not** (*circle your choice*) do something to help.

2. Abdominal thrusts should be directed in two directions, _____ and _____.

3. When giving abdominal thrusts, you should continue until either:

    a) _____ .

    b) _____ .

4. If choking may be a result of swelling of the airway, abdominal thrusts **will / will not** (*circle your choice*) work. You should get _____ as quickly as possible.

Found unconscious

5. As soon as you determine any casualty is unconscious, you should get _____ as quickly as possible.

6. You check for breathing and determine the casualty is NOT breathing. Your next step is to try to _____ into the casualty.

7. If you determine there is an obstruction, you will give _____ followed by a visual check in the mouth. Only remove an object if it's seen.

8. You **should / should not** (*circle your choice*) try breathing into the casualty again even if you do not find the blockage.

Special circumstances

9. If the casualty is pregnant, you should give _____ thrusts.

10. If the casualty is in a wheelchair, you must take them out of the wheelchair if they _____ .

11. If you are the casualty, and you are alone, you can try to dislodge the blockage using:

    a) _____ or

    b) _____ .

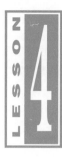

Objectives

- Apply the knowledge of cardiovascular disease
- Apply the knowledge of risk factors of cardiovascular disease
- Apply the knowledge of preventative health measures
- Apply the principles of first aid for cardiovascular emergencies
- Recognize angina/heart attack and provide first aid
- Recognize cardiac arrest
- Perform one rescuer CPR on an adult casualty
- Recognize stroke/TIA and provide first aid

Introduction

Cardiovascular disease kills more Canadians than any other cause of death. Some of these deaths could be prevented if appropriate first aid were given. Even more of these deaths could be prevented if individuals adopted a heart-healthy lifestyle that reduces the risk of cardiovascular disease.

Cardiovascular disease

Cardiovascular disease refers to disorders of the heart and blood vessels. High blood pressure and atherosclerosis are cardiovascular disorders. Over time, they can lead to cardiovascular emergencies such as angina, heart attack, congestive heart failure, transient ischemic attack, stroke and cardiac arrest. Each of these is described below.

High blood pressure

Blood pressure is the pressure of the blood against the inside walls of the blood vessels. Blood pressure goes up and down naturally. When a person is excited or emotionally stressed, blood pressure goes up, but it usually comes down once the excitement has passed. In some people, their blood pressure stays high all the time. This condition of constant high blood pressure is called **hypertension**. Over time, hypertension damages the tissues of the cardiovascular system. The walls of the blood vessels become thick and lose their elasticity and the heart becomes enlarged.

The changes caused by high blood pressure increase the risk of stroke, heart attack, kidney or eye problems. Unfortunately, hypertension does not always give warning signals—you may feel perfectly well but still have high blood pressure. This is why it is called the **silent killer**.

Narrowing of the arteries

Arteries are the blood vessels that carry blood away from the heart. They become diseased when fatty deposits build up inside them, making the passage for blood narrower. This process of fat deposition and narrowing of the arteries is called **atherosclerosis**. In the coronary arteries, which carry oxygenated blood to the heart, it is called **coronary artery disease**.

As an artery gets narrower, less and less blood gets through. When the artery gets too narrow, the tissues on the other side of the narrowing don't get enough oxygenated blood to function normally. Although the signs and symptoms of hardening of the arteries usually don't appear until middle age or later, atherosclerosis often begins in childhood.

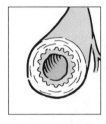

normal artery

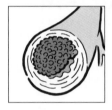

blocked artery

Angina

If one of the coronary arteries becomes hardened, the blood supply feeding that part of the heart muscle becomes limited. When the heart works harder and needs more blood (e.g. when you run for a bus or shovel snow), it can't get the oxygenated blood it needs through the narrowed coronary artery. This causes pain or discomfort in the chest which may spread to the neck, jaw, shoulders and arms. This pain is called **angina pectoris** (or "angina"). Angina pain doesn't usually last long, and goes away if the person rests and takes prescribed medication. Many people with angina live normally by taking medication that increases blood flow to the heart.

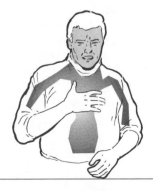

"You" – the Corner Stone to Survival

The Key Stones to Survival

CPR is often what comes to mind when people think of first aid for a heart attack or cardiac arrest. But CPR is only part of the picture. There are 4 keystones that provide direction to the first aider when helping someone with heart problems.

1. **early recognition** of a cardiovascular emergency

2. **early access** into the community emergency medical services (EMS) system. This means calling for help ... quickly

3. **early CPR** if required

4. **early defibrillation** if required (defibrillation is an electrical shock given to a quivering heart to make it beat properly again)

Each of the keystones is as important as the others. None of them alone will give the casualty the best chance for survival. Time is a vital ingredient. To give a casualty with no pulse a reasonable chance of survival, CPR must be started immediately followed by defibrillation as soon as possible. For both procedures, the sooner they happen, the better.

You, the first trained person on the scene, are responsible for initiating the sequence. You must recognize the cardiovascular emergency, call for medical help, start CPR if needed, and apply a defibrillator if trained. You play a crucial role as the "corner stone" to survival.

Don't worry, it's just indigestion.

I'm perfectly fit, I jog a mile a day. . . it's not my heart!

You watch, we'll wait a few minutes and the pain will go away.

A cup of tea and I'll be fine.

Early recognition and denial

The first of the keystones is "recognizing a cardiovascular emergency". This may be the toughest job you have to do. It's not easy to accept that someone is having a heart attack and could die very soon. This is especially true if the person is a family member or a close friend (family members and friends are often present during a heart attack). The person could still be talking to you and not *look* as if he is about to die. And perhaps the person is denying anything serious is happening, which often occurs.

On average, heart attack casualties take 4½ hours to get to a hospital from the time they first start feeling poorly. One reason for this is that it takes a long time to accept that something serious could be wrong.

It is this wasted time that prevents many lives from being saved. When someone complains of chest pain, you should consider it a serious problem—that's early recognition. The first thing you should do is call for medical help—that's "early access".

By getting the casualty to the hospital quickly, you will have given her the best chance for survival. If there is no serious problem, you will still have done the right thing and the casualty will have had a complete check-up. On the other hand, if there is a serious problem, you may have saved a life.

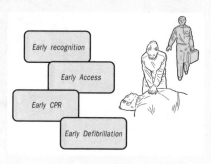

Early recognition
Early Access
Early CPR
Early Defibrillation

Heart attack

A heart attack happens when heart muscle tissue dies because its supply of oxygenated blood has been cut off. Usually, a blood clot gets stuck in a coronary artery that has been narrowed through atherosclerosis. The supply of blood is cut off and the heart tissue beyond the clot is starved of oxygen. A heart attack can feel just like angina, except the pain doesn't go away with rest and medication. If the heart attack damages the heart's electrical system, or if a lot of the heart muscle is affected, the heart may stop beating. This is cardiac arrest.

Doctors now have drugs to dissolve a blood clot, but they work best if given right away. This is why you have to get a casualty with a suspected heart attack to the hospital right away—the longer medical help is delayed, the more likely the heart will be damaged or stop beating. The medical term for a heart attack is **myocardial infarction** (my-o-car-dee-al in-fark-shun).

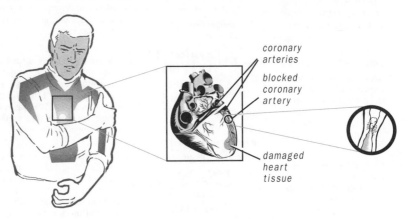

coronary
arteries

blocked
coronary
artery

damaged
heart
tissue

Signs and symptoms of angina and a heart attack

the pain may feel like:

- heaviness
- tightness
- squeezing
- pressure
- crushing
- indigestion
- aching jaw
- sore arms

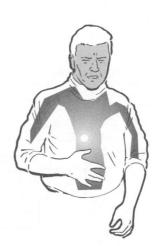

*a heart attack
can feel like
indigestion*

*other signs and symptoms
include:*

- denying anything is wrong
- fear
- pale skin
- nausea
- vomiting
- sweating
- shortness of breath
- fatigue
- shock
- unconsciousness
- cardiac arrest

First aid for angina/heart attack

A first aider may *understand* the difference between angina and a heart attack, but a first aider cannot *decide* whether a casualty is having angina pain or a heart attack—only a medical doctor can do this. For this reason, the first aid for angina and heart attack is the same.

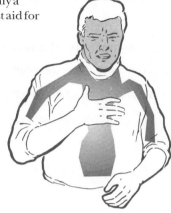

1 Begin ESM—do the scene survey.
   Ask the casualty questions to determine the scene history:

   "Can you show me where it hurts?"

   "Have you had this pain before?"

   "Do you have medication for this pain?"

2 Do a primary survey.

3 As soon as you recognize the signs and symptoms of angina/heart attack, call, or have a bystander call, for medical help. If you have to leave to call, place the casualty at rest (step 4) before you go.

4 Place the casualty at rest to reduce the work the heart has to do. The most comfortable position for the casualty is best.   In most cases, the semisitting position is best but this is not always the case. Let the casualty try what has helped before, but don't delay calling medical help while trying different positions to ease the pain.

5 Make the casualty comfortable—loosen tight clothing at the neck, chest and waist. Reassure the casualty to lessen fear and worry—these cause the heart to work harder.

6 Help the conscious casualty to take his prescribed medication. Follow the guidelines on page 4-6. If the casualty has no prescribed medication or there is no relief after the first dose of the prescribed medication, recommend that the conscious casualty chew 1 regular adult ASA tablet. Ask the casualty if he has any allergies to ASA or if a doctor has ever told him not to take ASA. Research has shown that the early administration of ASA can reduce the effects of a heart attack by as much as 20%.

7 If the casualty loses consciousness and stops breathing, start CPR.

Congestive heart failure

Heart failure means the heart can't pump blood effectively any more. Chronic heart disease or a previous heart attack may have led to this condition. Since the blood isn't pumped forward properly, it begins to back up in the lungs, causing breathing problems. The blood also backs up in the rest of the body and causes swelling, as in the ankles.

Signs and symptoms of heart failure

◆ inappropriate shortness of breath, especially when exercising

◆ difficulty breathing when lying flat

◆ blueness around the lips, fingernail beds, ears and other parts of the body

◆ swelling of the ankles

◆ coughing up frothy, pink fluid

First aid for heart failure

> Prevent medication errors by carefully checking the **five rights** for giving medicines—the **right medicine**, the **right person**, the **right amount**, the **right time**, the **right method**

1 Begin ESM—do the scene survey. Ask the casualty. questions to determine the scene history.

"Have you had breathing problems before?"

"Do you have a heart condition?"

"Do you have medication for this problem?

Do a primary survey.

2 Call for medical help.

3 Place the casualty at rest in a semisitting position and loosen tight clothing.

4 Reassure the casualty and monitor breathing closely.

Helping a casualty take medication

Only assist a casualty with medication if he or she is conscious and specifically asks for your help. Nitroglycerin tablets or sprays are common medications for relief of angina pain. Ask casualties if they use drugs to treat erectile dysfunction such as Viagra®.

If the person has taken any of these erectile dysfunction drugs do not assist the casualty to take nitroglycerin as this may cause a significant decrease in the person's blood pressure.

Ensure the medication is prescribed for this person. Spray the medication under the tongue or place the tablets under the tongue—they aren't to be swallowed or chewed.

The use of ASA is recommended. Nitroglycerin may be repeated, if needed, every 5-10 minutes to relieve pain, or until a maximum of three doses have been taken.

Stroke

If a blood clot blocks a narrowed artery in the brain and the part of the brain beyond the clot doesn't get the oxygen it needs, the brain tissue dies. This is called a **stroke** or **cerebrovascular accident** (CVA). A severe stroke can cause death. A less severe stroke may cause brain damage, which impairs certain body functions, depending on the part of the brain affected. In both heart attack and stroke, hardening of the arteries is the main cause. Over time, the arteries become narrowed and finally a clot blocks a narrowed artery. The difference between the heart attack and the stroke is the final resting place of the clot. A stroke can also be caused by a ruptured artery.

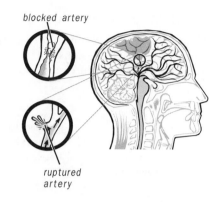

blocked artery

ruptured artery

A condition similar to a stroke is a **transient ischemic attack** (TIA). A TIA is caused by a lack of oxygen to part of the brain. It has the same signs and symptoms as a stroke. A TIA lasts from a few minutes to 24 hours and leaves no permanent brain damage. Although a TIA by itself is not life threatening, it is a warning sign that a stroke may follow. Advise anyone who has a TIA to get medical help.

Signs and symptoms of a stroke/TIA

The signs and symptoms of a stroke/TIA depend on what part of the brain is affected. Often, only one side of the body shows signs because only one side of the brain is affected. Remember F.A.S.T as a way to check for the signs of a stroke and to get immediate help.

*F*acial droop- one side of the face doesn't move as well as the other side

*A*rm drift- have casualty hold both arms out- one arm may not move or drifts down compared to the other arm

*S*peech- casualty slurs words, uses the incorrect words or is not able to speak

*T*ime- get immediate medical help- the earlier a stroke is treated the better the outcome

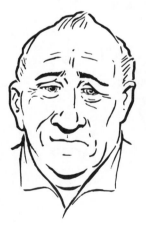

Casualties may complain of: **weakness** - sudden weakness, numbness or tingling in the face, arm or leg, **vision problems** - sudden loss of vision, particularly in one eye, or double vision, **headache** - sudden severe and unusual headache, **dizziness** - sudden loss of balance, especially with any of the above signs.

First aid for stroke/TIA

A first aider can't tell whether the casualty is having a stroke or a TIA, so the first aid is the same for both. If the signs and symptoms pass after a short while, suggesting the problem was a TIA, tell the casualty to see a doctor. A stroke could soon follow.

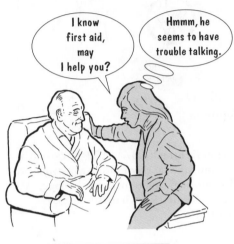

1 Begin ESM—do the scene survey. Ask the casualty questions to determine the scene history. Do a primary survey.

2 Call for medical help.

3 Place the casualty at rest in the most comfortable position—usually semisitting.

4 Give nothing by mouth. If the casualty is thirsty, moisten the lips with a wet cloth.

5 Protect the casualty from injury when they are lifted, moved or during convulsions.

6 Reassure the casualty and keep him warm.

7 If the casualty becomes semiconscious or unconscious, place them in the recovery position. If there is paralysis, place the paralyzed side up. This will reduce the chance of tissue or nerve damage to the affected side.

8 If casualty becomes unresponsive and breathing stops start CPR.

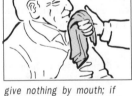

give nothing by mouth; if the casualty complains of thirst, moisten lips with a wet cloth

Which side is paralyzed?

. . . .

If the casualty becomes unconscious, it may be hard to tell if there is any paralysis. The mouth and cheek on the paralyzed side may droop more than the non-paralyzed side—the face may look "crooked."

If you can, place the casualty in the recovery position with the paralyzed side up.

paralyzed side up

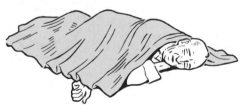

if the casualty becomes semiconscious or unconscious, place them in the recovery position

Cardiac arrest

When the heart stops pumping, it is in **cardiac arrest**. A cardiac arrest can happen suddenly or may follow a period of stopped or ineffective breathing, when much of the oxygen in the body is used up. A heart attack causes cardiac arrest when so much heart tissue is damaged that it can't pump blood anymore. Other reasons for cardiac arrest include severe injuries, electrical shock, drug overdose, drowning, suffocation and stroke. When a person's heart has stopped, they are considered **clinically dead** even though they may still be resuscitated. The first aid for cardiac arrest is cardiopulmonary resuscitation (CPR) as described in the sequence below.

Cardiopulmonary resuscitation (CPR)

CPR is two basic life support skills put together—artificial respiration and artificial circulation. Artificial respiration provides oxygen to the lungs. Artificial circulation causes blood to flow through the body, but flows only enough to give a person a chance for survival. The purpose of CPR is to circulate oxygenated blood to the brain and other organs until either the heart starts beating, or medical help takes over.

The CPR sequence follows from the scene survey and primary survey outlined in Lesson 1, *Emergency Scene Management.*

When you find an unresponsive casualty, send for help immediately (scene survey). Then, start the primary survey by opening the airway and checking for normal breathing. If there is no breathing, give two breaths.

If the breaths go in you will see the chest rise. Feel for a pulse at the side of the neck. If you cannot feel a pulse or if you are unsure, CPR compressions are needed.

Next begin CPR. If an automated external defibrillator (AED) is available, use as soon as possible.

Ages in CPR

In CPR, AR and first aid for choking, the following age guidelines are used:

◆ infant = under 1 year old

◆ child = 1 year of age to 8 years of age

◆ adult = over 8 years of age

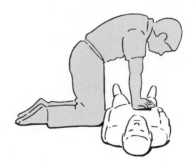

CPR – adult casualty

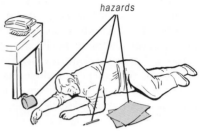

You arrive at a scene…an unconscious adult (over 8 years of age) is lying on the floor…

1   Begin ESM—start the scene survey.

- -

2   Assess responsiveness.

ask the casualty if they are O.K. Assess any response

gently tap the shoulders

Are you O.K.?

If there is no response, go to step 3.

- -

3   Send or go for medical help and an AED if available. If you are alone, see page 1-9 for information on when to go for medical help.

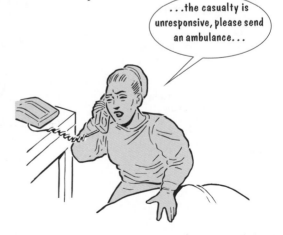

…the casualty is unresponsive, please send an ambulance…

4 Place the casualty face up, protecting the head and neck during any movement. Open the airway by tilting the head and lifting the jaw.

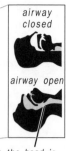

airway closed

airway open

to open the airway push backward on the forehead and lift the chin

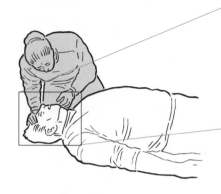

when the head is tilted back, the tongue is lifted off the back of the throat, opening the airway

5 Check for normal breathing for up to 10 seconds.

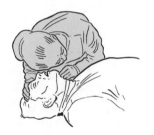

keep the head tilted

place your ear just above the casualty's nose and mouth

look. . . for chest movement

listen. . . for sounds of breathing

feel. . . for breath on your cheek

Agonal Breathing

Agonal breathing may be present in cardiac arrest casualties. Casualties will have gasping with no regular pattern or depth. Do not confuse this with regular breathing.

If there is no breathing, go to step 6.

6 Breathe into the casualty twice. For an adult casualty, each breath should take about 1 second. Use enough air to make the chest rise.

if

take a normal breath and seal your mouth around the casualty's mouth

pinch the nostrils

blow in and watch for the chest to rise

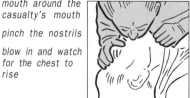

move your mouth away and release the nostrils to allow the air to escape

look for the chest to fall, listen for air sounds and feel for air being exhaled against your cheek

give another breath and go to step 7

If the chest doesn't rise when you blow:

♦ reopen the airway by tilting the head & lifting the jaw

♦ pinch the nose again

♦ make a better seal around the mouth

♦ try blowing again

If the chest still doesn't rise, give first aid for choking—see page 3-6.

7   Check for a pulse at the side of the neck. Be aware that pulses can be hard to find. If there is no pulse or you are unsure, begin CPR

. . . .

8   Start CPR.

Make sure the casualty is on a firm, flat surface and position your hands on the chest for chest compressions.

kneel so your hands can be placed mid-chest

place 2 hands in the centre of the upper chest and give 30 compressions

use the hand position you find easiest

- fingers interlocked
- fingers straight
- holding wrist

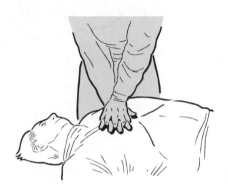

If an AED is available and you or another person is trained to use the machine, attach device as soon as possible and follow the voice prompts from the machine.

With your hands in place, position your shoulders directly over your hands and keep your elbows locked.

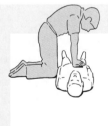

9 Give 30 compressions.. **Push hard, push fast.**

Actual depth

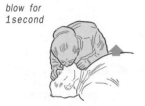

0 cm

1 and 2 and 3 and 4 and 5 and 6 and 7 and 8 and 9 and 10...

3.8 cm (1½ in)

depress the chest 3.8 to 5 cm

5 cm (2 in)

depress and release the chest rhythmically

press the heels of the hands straight down on the breastbone

the pressure and release phases take the same time

release pressure and completely remove your weight at the top of each compression to allow chest to return to the resting position after each compression.

give compressions at a rate of 100 per minute

count compressions out loud to keep track of how many you have given, and to help keep a steady rhythm

... and two ventilations—this is one **cycle** of 30:2 (30 compressions to 2 ventilations).

blow for 1 second

watch for the chest to fall, feel air being exhaled

blow for 1 second

10 Continue compressions and ventilations in the ratio of 30:2 starting with compressions. Continue CPR until either:

◆ an AED is applied,

◆ the casualty starts to respond,

◆ another first aider takes over,

◆ medical help takes over ,

◆ you are exhausted and cannot continue.

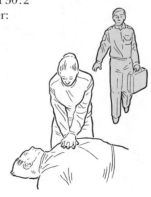

How to take over
CPR from another rescuer

• •

CPR can be tiring. In order to maintain the most effective compressions it is recommended that rescuers switch after every 5 cycles of compressions and ventilations (approx 2 minutes).

1

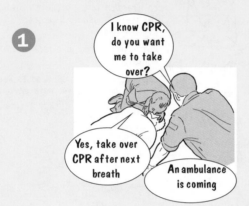

ask if you can help

find out if medical help has been called

2

give 30 compressions

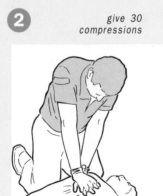

3

give two breaths

continue CPR with cycles of 30 compressions and two ventilations

don't use the same face shield as the first rescuer

Cardiovascular Emergencies - Activity

· ·

· · · · · · · · · · **Angina and heart attack** · · · · · · · · · ·

1. _Cardiovascular_ refers to disorders of the heart and blood vessels.

2. Narrowing of arteries is caused by a build up of _fatty deposits_ on the inside lining. This results in reduced _oxygen_ to the tissues on the other side of the narrowing.

3. _Angina_ refers to the pain or discomfort in the chest which may spread to the neck, jaw, shoulders and arms. This pain does not last long and goes away if the person rests and takes prescribed medication.

4. Many people with angina live normally by taking _medication_ that increases blood flow to the heart.

5. A _heart attack_ happens when the heart muscle dies because its supply of oxygenated blood has been cut off.

6. Signs and symptoms of angina and heart attack include:

   a) _____

   b) _____

   c) _____

   d) _____ .

7. If you suspect someone is having a heart attack, it is important to get _medical help_ right away.

8. If you suspect a casualty is having angina or a heart attack,

   a) place the casualty _at rest_ to reduce the work of the heart.

   b) Help the casualty to take _medication_, if appropriate.

   c) Give _CPR_ if he loses consciousness, stops breathing and you cannot feel a pulse.

Cardiovascular Emergencies - Activity

Stroke/TIA

9. A ___stroke___ results where a blood clot blocks a narrowed artery in the brain and the part of the brain beyond the clot doesn't get the oxygen it needs, the brain tissue dies.

10. A condition similar to a stroke is a ___TIA___. It has the same signs and symptoms as a stroke and only lasts from a few minutes to 24 hours, *usually* leaving no permanent brain damage.

11. A TIA is a warning sign that a ___stroke___ may follow.

12. Signs and symptoms of a stroke or TIA include:

    a) _____
    b) _____   4-7
    c) _____
    d) _____ .

Cardiopulmonary resuscitation

13. CPR is two basic life support skills put together — ___Artificial respiration___ and ___Chest compression___.

14. If you find an unresponsive casualty, send for ___medical help___ immediately and an ___AED___ if available.

15 If the casualty is unresponsive, not breathing normally, and does not have a pulse begin CPR at a ratio of ___30___ compressions to ___2___ breaths.

16. Continue CPR until either:

    a) ___we are relieved___
    b) ___an AED is applied___
    c) ___signs of life___
    d) ___we are too exhausted___ .

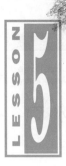

Objectives

◆ Use dressings and bandages in first aid procedures

◆ Recognize major wounds

◆ Recognize severe external and internal bleeding

◆ Provide first aid for wounds with severe external bleeding

◆ Provide first aid for amputations and care for amputated tissue

◆ Recognize inadequate circulation to the extremities and provide the appropriate first aid

◆ Provide first aid for internal bleeding

Wounds and bleeding

A **wound** is any break in the soft tissues of the body. It usually results in bleeding and may allow germs to enter the body. **Bleeding** is the escape of blood from the blood vessels into surrounding tissues, body cavities or out of the body. The soft tissues of the body are the most susceptible to injury, resulting in wounds and bleeding.

A wound can be either open or closed:

◆ **open wound**—there is a break in the outer layer of the skin that results in bleeding and may permit germs to enter the body, causing infection

◆ **closed wound**—there is no break in the outer layer of skin so there is no external bleeding (but there will be internal bleeding which may be severe) and the risk of infection is low (except in internal abdominal injuries where the risk of infection is high)

The different types of open and closed wounds to soft tissues are given in the table on the next page. When someone is injured, recognizing the type of wound helps to give appropriate first aid.

The aim in the care of wounds is to stop the bleeding and prevent infection. Although some bleeding may help to wash contamination from the wound, excessive blood flow must be stopped quickly to minimize shock.

Bleeding

Bleeding is the escape of blood from the blood vessels. In **external bleeding**, blood escapes the body through a surface wound—you can see external bleeding. In **internal bleeding**, blood escapes from tissues inside the body—you don't usually see internal bleeding. Also, bleeding is either **arterial**, which is bleeding from the arteries, or **venous**, which is bleeding from the veins.

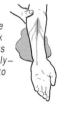

*in **arterial** bleeding, the blood is bright red and spurts with each heartbeat—arterial bleeding is serious and often hard to control*

*in **venous** bleeding, the blood is dark red and flows more steadily—it is easier to stop than arterial bleeding*

Contusions or bruises	Abrasions or scrapes	Incisions	Lacerations	Puncture wounds	Avulsions & Amputations

Contusions or bruises are closed wounds usually caused by a fall or a blow from something blunt. The tissues under the skin are damaged and bleed into surrounding tissues, causing discolouration.

Because there is no break in the skin, there is little chance of infection. A bruise may be a sign of a deeper, more serious injury or illness.

Abrasions or scrapes are open wounds where the outer protective layer of skin and the tiny underlying blood vessels are exposed, but the deeper layer of the skin is still intact.

Abrasions are usually due to the skin being scraped across a hard surface (rug burns, road rash).

Abrasions do not bleed very much but can be very painful. The risk of infection from dirt and other particles that may be in the wound is high.

Incisions are clean cuts in soft tissue caused by something sharp such as a knife. These wounds may not be as dirty as abrasions, but they may contain fragments of glass or other material.

Lacerations are tears in the skin and underlying tissue. The edges of the wound are jagged and irregular, and dirt is likely to be present, increasing the risk of infection.

Lacerations are often caused by machinery, barbed wire or the claws of an animal.

Puncture wounds are open wounds caused by blunt or pointed instruments, such as knives, nails or an animal's teeth.

The wound may have a small opening, but often penetrates deep into the tissue. There may be contamination deep in the wound and internal organs may be damaged.

Avulsions are injuries that leave a piece of skin or other tissue either partially or completely torn away from the body.

Amputations involve partial or complete loss of a body part and are usually caused by machinery or cutting tools.

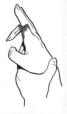

Gunshot wounds are a special type of wound. The entry wound is often small, and may have burns around it. Sometimes there is an exit wound as well, which is usually larger than the entry wound. Because the bullet may bounce around inside the body, the exit wound may not be directly across from the entry wound.

Signs and symptoms of bleeding

The most obvious sign of external bleeding is blood. You do not always see blood with internal bleeding. General signs and symptoms of bleeding vary depending on how much blood is lost. Severe blood loss will result in the following signs and symptoms of shock:

◆ pale, cool and clammy skin

◆ rapid pulse, gradually becoming weaker

◆ faintness, dizziness, thirst and nausea

◆ restlessness and apprehension

◆ shallow breathing, yawning, sighing and gasping for air

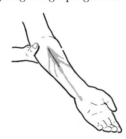

Principles of controlling bleeding

The body has natural defences against bleeding. Damaged blood vessels constrict to reduce blood flow and blood pressure drops as bleeding continues. These factors result in reduced force of blood flow. Blood will clot as it is exposed to air, forming a seal at the wound. Even so, the first aider should try to stop all bleeding as soon as possible, following the ABC priorities.

Steps to control bleeding

Direct pressure—apply pressure directly to the wound to stop blood flow and allow clots to form. When bleeding is controlled, keep the pressure on the wound with dressings and bandages.

Rest—place the casualty at rest to reduce the pulse rate.

Minor cuts and scrapes that cause slight bleeding are easily controlled with pressure, and rest. Severe bleeding must be brought under control quickly to prevent further blood loss and to slow the progress of shock.

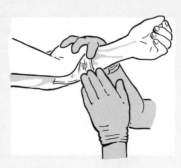

Dressings and bandages

Dressings and bandages are the basic tools of first aid. They are essential for wound care and for the care of injuries to bones, joints and muscles. You should know how to use commercially prepared dressings and bandages, and also be ready to improvise with materials on hand at the emergency scene. Knowing what makes a good dressing and bandage helps you do this.

Dressings

A dressing is a protective covering put on a wound to help control bleeding, absorb blood from the wound, and prevent further contamination. A dressing should be:

- ◆ sterile, or as clean as possible

- ◆ large enough to completely cover the wound

- ◆ highly absorbent to keep the wound dry

- ◆ compressible, thick and soft—especially for severe bleeding so that pressure is applied evenly over the wound

- ◆ non-stick and lint-free to reduce the possibility of sticking to the wound—gauze, cotton and linen make good dressings; wool or other fluffy materials make poor dressings

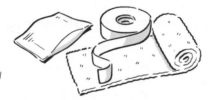

commercial dressings

Dressings are available in a variety of sizes and designs. The dressings used most often in first aid are:

- ◆ *adhesive dressings*—prepared sterile gauze dressings with their own adhesive strips. They are sealed in a paper or plastic covering and are available in various sizes and shapes, according to their intended use. They are often used for minor wounds with little bleeding

- ◆ *gauze dressings*—in varying sizes, folded and packaged individually or in large numbers—packaged gauze is usually sterile

- ◆ *pressure dressings*—sterile dressings of gauze and other absorbent material, usually with an attached roller bandage. They are used to apply pressure to a wound with severe bleeding

◆ *improvised dressings*—prepared from lint-free sterile or clean material, preferably white. They may be made from a towel, a sheet, a pillow slip or any other clean absorbent material such as a sanitary pad. Plastic wrap or the wrapping from a sterile dressing can be used as an airtight dressing for penetrating wounds of the chest

Follow the guidelines below for putting on dressings:

◆ prevent further contamination as much as you can—use the cleanest material available as dressings, and wear gloves or wash your hands before handling them—see page 1-5 for more on preventing further contamination

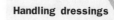

improvised dressings

◆ extend the dressing beyond the edges of the wound to completely cover it

◆ if blood soaks through a dressing, leave it in place and cover with more dressings

◆ secure a dressing with tape or bandages

Bandages

A bandage is any material that is used to hold a dressing in place, maintain pressure over a wound, support a limb or joint, immobilize parts of the body or secure a splint. Bandages may be commercially prepared or improvised.

When using bandages, remember to:

◆ apply them firmly to make sure bleeding is controlled or immobilization is achieved

◆ check the circulation beyond the bandage frequently to ensure the bandage is not too tight

◆ use your bandages only as bandages, not as padding or dressings, when other materials are available—you may need all your bandages for other injuries

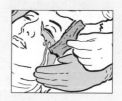

Handling dressings
. . . .
When handling dressings, never touch the surface that will touch the wound. Always handle a dressing from the outer side.

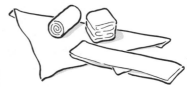

commercial bandages

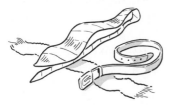

improvised bandages

The triangular bandage

One of the most versatile prepared or improvised bandages is the triangular bandage. It is made by cutting a one-metre square of linen or cotton on the diagonal, producing two triangles. Triangular bandages can be improvised from sheets, garbage bags, canvas, etc. The parts of the triangular bandage, identified for ease of instruction, are:

A triangular bandage may be used:

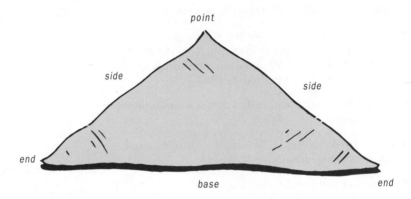

- ◆ as a **whole cloth**—opened to its fullest extent, as a sling or to hold a large dressing in place

- ◆ as a **broad bandage**—to hold splints in place or to apply pressure evenly over a large area

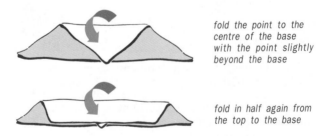

fold the point to the centre of the base with the point slightly beyond the base

fold in half again from the top to the base

- ◆ as a **narrow bandage**—to secure dressings or splints or to immobilize ankles and feet in a figure-8

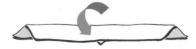

fold a broad bandage in half again from the top to the base

◆ as a **ring pad**—to control bleeding when pressure cannot be applied directly to the wound, as in the case of a short embedded object. Prepare a ring pad for your first aid kit, ready for use

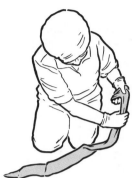

make a narrow bandage

form a loop around one hand by wrapping one end of the bandage twice around four fingers

pass the loose end through the loop and wrap it around and around until the entire bandage is used up and a firm ring is

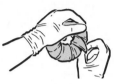

made—this is a ring pad

to make a ring pad with a larger loop, tie two narrow bandages together

Reef knot—the knot of choice

The reef knot is the best knot for tying bandages and slings because:

◆ it lies flat, making it more comfortable than other knots

◆ it doesn't slip

◆ it is easy to untie

To tie a reef knot:

◆ take one end of a bandage in each hand

◆ lay the end from the right hand over the one from the left hand and pass it under to form a half-knot. This will transfer the ends from one hand to the other

◆ the end now in the left hand should be laid over the one from the right and passed under to form another half-knot. The finished knot looks like two inter-twined loops

◆ tighten by pulling one loop against the other or by pulling only on the ends

Place knots so they do not cause discomfort by pressing on skin or bone, particularly at the site of a fracture or at the neck, when tying a sling.

If the knot is uncomfortable, place soft material underneath as padding.

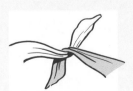

right over left, and under

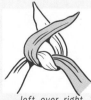

left over right and under

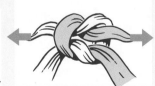

pull the ends to tighten

First aid for severe external bleeding

The principles of first aid for bleeding and preventing further contamination are on page 5-3. The following sequence shows the principles being used.

1   Begin ESM—do a scene survey. Assess the mechanism of injury. If you suspect a head or spinal injury, steady and support the head and neck before continuing.

. . . .

2   Do a primary survey and give first aid for life-threatening injuries.

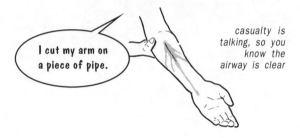

I cut my arm on a piece of pipe.

casualty is talking, so you know the airway is clear

. . . .

3   To control severe bleeding, apply direct pressure to the wound as quickly as possible. If the wound is large and wide open, you may have to bring the edges of the wound together first.

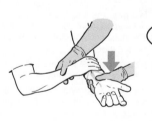

How is your breathing?

the first aider shows the casualty how to apply direct pressure to control the bleeding

. . . .

4 Place the casualty at rest—this will further reduce blood flow and will reduce the risk of injury if the casualty becomes dizzy or faints.

5 Quickly replace the casualty's hand with dressings (preferably sterile) and continue direct pressure over the dressings.

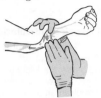

6 Once bleeding is under control, continue the primary survey, looking for other life-threatening injuries. Give life-saving first aid as needed.

7 Before bandaging the wound, check circulation below the injury.

 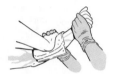

check the temperature and colour of the fingers and use the nailbed test—see page 5-10

8 Bandage the dressing in place.

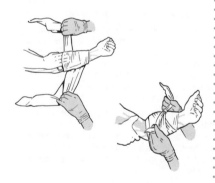

9 Check the circulation below the injury and compare it with the other side. If it is worse than it was before the injury was bandaged, loosen the bandage just enough to improve circulation.

10 Give ongoing casualty care, including first aid to minimize shock—see page 2-3.

If the dressings become blood-soaked...

... don't remove them—add more dressings and continue pressure. Removing the blood-soaked dressings may disturb blood clots and expose the wound to further contamination.

Checking
circulation below an injury

Causes of impaired circulation

Certain injuries and first aid procedures may impair (reduce or cut off) circulation to the tissue below the injury (called *distal* circulation). A joint injury or fracture could pinch an artery and restrict the flow of blood to the limb. Bandages tied too tightly will impair distal circulation. Sometimes, a bandage is not too tight when it is put on but as the injury swells, the bandage becomes too tight, impairing circulation.

the nailbed test

How to monitor circulation

For each of the methods below, check both the injured side and the uninjured side of the casualty. If circulation is not impaired, both sides will be the same. Monitor circulation below the injury by:

♦ checking skin colour—if the skin does not have full colour, circulation may be impaired

♦ checking skin temperature—if the skin temperature feels cold, especially if it is colder than the uninjured side, circulation may be impaired

♦ checking for a pulse - in an arm injury, check for a pulse at the wrist (if trained)

♦ doing the nailbed test—press on a fingernail or toenail until the nailbed turns white, and then release it. Note how long it takes for normal colour to return. If it returns quickly, blood flow is unrestricted. If it stays white, or if the colour returns slowly, circulation may be impaired

When the injury is on the arm, expose the hands and fingers to check circulation. When the injury is on the leg and there is no reason to remove the shoe, check circulation by placing fingers inside the sock along the side of the foot.

Effects of impaired circulation

If oxygenated blood does not reach the tissues below the injury, there may be tissue damage that could lead to loss of the limb. Check circulation below an injury before tying any bandages. Check again after tying bandages. If circulation is impaired, take steps to improve it.

Improving impaired circulation

To improve impaired circulation, loosen tight bandages. If circulation doesn't improve and medical help will be delayed, try moving the limb to restore circulation. By moving the limb, you will hopefully relieve any pressure on blood vessels. If possible, move the limb towards its natural position. Only **move the limb as much as the casualty will let you, or as far as you can without resistance.** Resecure the limb and recheck circulation.

Keep monitoring circulation until medical help takes over. If circulation remains impaired, medical help is urgently needed.

Amputations

An amputation is when a part of the body, such as a toe, foot or leg, has been partly or completely cut off. When this happens, you must control the bleeding from the wound, care for the amputated tissue and get medical help. The first aid for both a completely amputated hand and a partly amputated finger is shown below.

First aid for amputations

1   Begin ESM—do a scene survey. Do a primary survey and give first aid for life-threatening injuries. In this case, there is severe bleeding from an amputation.

. . . .

2   Control the bleeding—apply direct pressure to the wound.

. . . .

3   Send for medical help and give ongoing casualty care to the casualty, including first aid for shock.

completely amputated hand

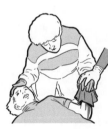

stop the bleeding:
- apply direct pressure
- place the casualty at rest & bandage the dressings in place

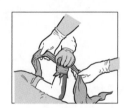

partly amputated finger

reposition a partly amputated part to its normal position

apply direct pressure and cover the area with thick sterile gauze that is moistened, if possible

bandage in position

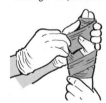

Priorities

. . . .

Always give life-saving first aid to the casualty before giving care to the amputated part.

4   Care for the amputated tissue—completely or partly amputated parts must be preserved, regardless of their condition, and taken to medical help with the casualty. It may be possible to reattach the part—and with the proper care of the part, the chances are even better. Care for the amputated part as follows:

. . . .

5   Keep the amputated part in a shaded, cool place and get the casualty and the amputated part to medical help as soon as possible.

wrap the amputated part in a clean, moist dressing—if you can't moisten the dressing, a dry dressing will do

gauze dresssing

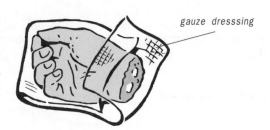

put the amputated part in a clean, watertight plastic bag and seal it

put this bag in a second plastic bag or container partly filled with crushed ice

attach a record of the date and time this was done and send this package with the casualty to medical help

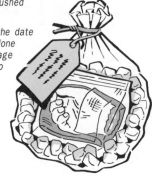

 Do not. . .

. . . try to clean an amputated part. Do not use any antiseptic solutions.

Preventing further contamination

All open wounds are contaminated to some degree. From the moment of injury, there is risk of infection that continues until the wound is completely healed. Stopping bleeding is your priority, but do it using the cleanest materials available.

Minor wound care

Follow the principles listed below for cleaning a wound. Tell the casualty to seek medical help if signs of infection appear later (see info box below).

◆ wash your hands with soap and water and put on gloves if available

◆ do not cough or breathe directly over the wound

◆ fully expose the wound but don't touch it

◆ gently wash loose material from the surface of the wound. Wash and dry the surrounding skin with clean dressings, wiping away from the wound. An antibiotic cream (preferably triple antibiotic) can be used on superficial wound and abrasions

◆ cover the wound promptly with a sterile dressing. Tape the dressing in place

◆ remove and dispose of gloves in an appropriate manner and wash your hands and any other skin area that may have been in contact with the casualty's blood

Tetanus Infection

Any wound may be contaminated by spores that cause tetanus, a potentially fatal disease characterized by muscle spasms. Tetanus is commonly referred to as "lockjaw."

Deep wounds, especially those caused by animal bites or those that may have been contaminated by soil, dust or animal feces, are at high risk of tetanus infection. Advise a casualty with this type of wound to get medical help.

Recognizing internal bleeding

Internal bleeding may not be easy to recognize—a casualty can bleed to death without any blood being seen. Suspect internal bleeding if:

◆ the casualty received a severe blow or a penetrating injury to the chest, neck, abdomen or groin

◆ there are major limb fractures such as a fractured upper leg or pelvis

Wound infection

Any wound that becomes infected should be seen by a doctor. Recognize infection in a wound when the wound:

◆ becomes more painful

◆ becomes red and perhaps swollen

◆ feels warmer than the surrounding area

◆ shows the presence of pus (whitish fluid)

Signs of internal bleeding

You may recognize internal bleeding by one or more of the following characteristic signs. Blood is:

◆ coming from the ear canal or the nose, or it may appear as a bloodshot eye or black eye (bleeding inside the head)

◆ coughed up and looks bright red and frothy (bleeding into the lungs)

◆ seen in vomitus either as bright red, or brown like coffee grounds

◆ seen in the stools, and looks either black and tarry (bleeding into the upper bowel), or its normal red colour (bleeding into the lower bowel)

◆ seen in the urine as a red or smoky brown colour (bleeding into the urinary tract)

First aid for severe, internal bleeding

As a first aider, you can do very little to control internal bleeding. Give first aid to minimize shock and get medical help as quickly as you can.

If internal bleeding is severe, signs of shock will be present.

1 Begin ESM—do a scene survey.

. . . .

2 Do a primary survey and give first aid for life-threatening injuries. In this case, you suspect severe internal bleeding.

If the casualty is conscious, place them at rest on their back with the feet and legs raised to about 30 cm (12 in).

If the casualty is unconscious, place them in the recovery position.

if the mechanism of injury suggests a severe blow to the body, look further for signs of internal bleeding

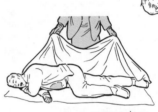

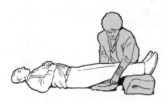

conscious casualty in shock position

unconscious casualty in recovery position

. . . .

3 Send or go for medical help.

. . . .

4 Give ongoing casualty care. Do not give the casualty anything by mouth. If they complain of thirst, moisten their lips with a wet cloth. Make the casualty comfortable—loosen all tight clothing at the neck, chest and waist. Keep the casualty warm and protected from extreme temperatures.

Monitor the casualty often. When medical help takes over, make sure you tell them you suspect internal bleeding.

⚠ Keep track of. . .

. . . .

. . . any changes in level of consciousness, breathing, pulse and skin temperature. Relay this information to medical help.

Severe Bleeding - Activity

Dressings and bandages

1. A _____ is a protective covering used to control bleeding.

2. A bandage is any material used to:

   a) _____

   b) _____

   c) _____

   d) _____

   e) _____ .

3. The _____ bandage is the most versatile of either prepared or improvised. It can be used in four formats, as:

   a) _____

   b) _____

   c) _____

   d) _____ .

4. Examples of improvised dressings include:_____.

   Examples of improvised bandages include:_____.

Severe external bleeding

5. The principles of wound management (controlling bleeding) are:

   a) _____

   b) _____ .

6. You should check for adequate _____ in a limb both before and after bandaging a wound.

7. The priorities for first aid in the case of an amputation are:

   a) _____

   b) _____

   c) _____ .

Severe Bleeding - Activity

· ·

8. Signs of infection in a wound include:

    a) _____

    b) _____

    c) _____

    d) _____ .

9. _____ is a potentially fatal disease characterized by muscle spasms. This condition can result from animal bites or other wounds exposed to contaminants.

10. Steps you can take to reduce the risk of infection include:

    a) _____

    b) _____

    c) _____ .

· · · · · · · · · · **Severe internal bleeding** · · · · · · · · · ·

11. Signs of internal bleeding include:

    a) _____

    b) _____

    c) _____

    d) _____

    e) _____ .

12. The conscious casualty with signs of internal bleeding should be positioned in a _____ position.

    The unconscious cacasualty with signs of internal bleeding should be positioned in a _____ position.

13. In cases of suspected internal bleeding, get _____ as quickly as possible.

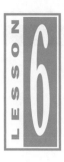

LESSON 6

Diabetic emergency

In a healthy person, the body produces the **insulin** needed to allow cells to take up sugar and convert the sugar into energy. **Diabetes** is a condition in which there is either not enough insulin in the blood or there is enough insulin but the cells cannot use the insulin properly. As a result, sugar builds up in the blood, and the cells don't get the energy they need. A person with diabetes takes medication by mouth or injection, and carefully controls what they eat (the source of energy) and their level of exercise (the use of energy). A diabetic emergency occurs when there is too much or too little insulin in the blood.

hypoglycemia –not enough sugar, too much insulin

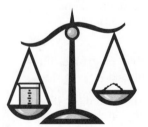

hyperglycemia– too much sugar, not enough insulin

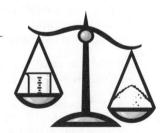

There are two kinds of diabetic emergency—**hypoglycemia** and **hyperglycemia**. The signs and symptoms for each are listed in the table on the following page, along with the possible causes. As a first aider, it is not important to know the type of diabetic emergency—follow the first aid on the next page.

What is important is that you recognize the casualty's condition as an emergency and get medical help quickly.

Causes, signs and symptoms of diabetic emergencies

	hypoglycemia (needs sugar)	hyperglycemia (needs insulin)
time to develop	develops very quickly	develops over hours or days
possible cause	– took too much insulin – not eaten enough, or vomited – more exercise than usual	– did not take enough insulin – eating too much food – less exercise than usual – casualty has an ongoing illness and her body needs more insulin
pulse	strong rapid	weak and rapid
breathing	shallow	deep and sighing
skin condition	sweaty, pale and cold	flushed, dry and warm
level of consc.	faintness to unconscious	drowsy, becoming unconscious
other signs and symptoms	– headache – confused, irritable and aggressive – trembling, staggering – difficulty speaking	– thirsty, then nausea and vomiting – frequent urination – breath has a nail polish smell

First aid for diabetic emergencies

The aim of first aid in a diabetic emergency is to keep the casualty's condition from getting worse while you get medical help.

1   Begin ESM—do a scene survey. If the casualty is unresponsive, get medical help immediately. If you are alone—see page 1-9.

2   Do a primary survey and give first aid for the ABCs.

3   If the casualty is unconscious, place them into the recovery position and monitor the ABCs until medical help takes over. The casualty may be wearing a medical alert device that will give you more information about their condition.

look for a medical alert device at the neck, wrist or ankle

If the casualty is conscious, ask what is wrong. They may be able to tell you, or they may be confused.

◆ if the casualty can tell you what they need, or if you can tell by the signs and symptoms, help them take what is needed—this is usually sugar

◆ if the casualty is confused about what is needed, give them something sweet to eat or drink—sugar may help, and if it doesn't, it won't make the casualty any worse

sweeten a drink with 30 ml (2 tablespoons) of sugar or something else sweet, like apple or orange juice (no diet soft drinks)

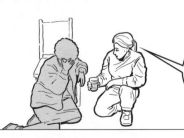

I know you're not sure what's wrong, but drinking this may help and it won't hurt.

4   Give ongoing casualty care. Send for medical help if you have not done so already.

if the casualty is conscious and very weak, place them in the position of most comfort, which may be the shock position

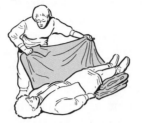

Seizures and convulsions

A **seizure** is caused by abnormal electrical activity in the brain. In a **partial seizure**, only part of the brain is affected. The person may experience a tingling or twitching in one area of the body. In a **generalized seizure**, the whole brain is affected—the person loses consciousness and may have convulsions. A **convulsion** is an abnormal muscle contraction, or series of muscle contractions, that the person cannot control.

Epilepsy is a disorder of the nervous system characterized by seizures. Many people with seizure disorders like epilepsy take medication to control the condition. Other causes of seizures include:

- head injury
- brain infection
- a high fever in infants and children
- stroke
- drug overdose

With epilepsy, the person may feel that a seizure is about to occur because of a brief sensation they experience, called an **aura**. The aura, which may be a hallucinated sound, smell, or a feeling of movement in the body, is felt just before the seizure. A major seizure can come on very suddenly, but seldom lasts longer than three minutes. After the seizure, the person may not remember what happened. They may appear dazed and confused, and feel exhausted and sleepy.

Signs and symptoms of a generalized seizure

- a sudden cry, stiffening of the body and loss of consciousness causing the person to fall
- noisy breathing and frothy saliva at the mouth
- the body jerks
- breathing may stop or be irregular for a minute —the casualty may turn blue
- loss of bladder and bowel control

A typical generalized seizure . . .
. . . .
. . . has two major phases:

The **"tonic"** phase:

- a sudden loss of consciousness causing the person to fall. The person's body becomes rigid for up to a minute during which the face and neck may turn bluish.

The **"clonic"** phase:

- convulsions occur, breathing is noisy, frothy saliva may appear around the mouth and the teeth may grind.

When the seizure is over, the muscles gradually relax and the person regains consciousness.

First aid for a seizure or convulsion

First aid for a seizure aims to protect the casualty from injury during convulsions and to keep the airway open while the casualty is unconscious.

1 Begin ESM—do a scene survey (see page 1-12). Make the area safe—clear away hard or sharp objects that could cause injury. Clear onlookers away to ensure the casualty's privacy.

turning the casualty to the side allows for drainage of fluids, and keeps the tongue from falling back and blocking the airway

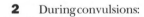

2 During convulsions:

- don't restrict the casualty's movements. Gently guide them, if necessary, to protect from injury

- carefully loosen tight clothing, especially around the neck

- place something soft under the head

- **do not** try to put anything in the mouth, between the teeth or to hold the tongue

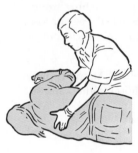

3 After convulsions:

after convulsions, place the unconscious casualty into the recovery position

- assess responsiveness and do a primary survey. Place the unconscious casualty into the recovery position— wipe away any fluids from the mouth and nose

- do a secondary survey to see if the casualty was injured during the seizure (although it is rare, injury is possible)—give first aid for any injuries

- give ongoing casualty care, monitoring breathing, keeping the casualty warm and allowing them to rest (they may need up to an hour)

- don't give the casualty any liquids during or immediately after a seizure

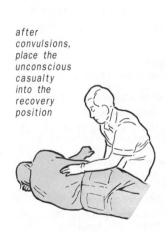

Call for medical help if:

- the casualty is unconscious for more than five minutes, or has a second seizure within a few minutes

- this is the person's first seizure or the cause of the seizure is unknown (ask the casualty when they regain consciousness)

Fever emergencies in infants and children

A rapid rise in temperature to 40°C (104°F) or higher can cause convulsions in infants and children. A fever emergency is when the temperature, taken in the armpit, is:

◆ 38°C (100.5°F) or higher for an infant

◆ 40°C (104°F) or higher for a child

First aid for a fever emergency in an infant or child

1   Begin ESM—do a scene survey.

2   Advise the parent/caregiver to call the doctor immediately and follow her advice. If the doctor can't be reached, advise the parent/caregiver to give children's ibuprofen or acetaminophen, not ASA—see warning below) according to the directions on the label. This should bring down the child's temperature.

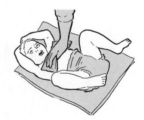

sponge the child with lukewarm water for 20 minutes

3   If fully conscious, encourage the child to drink fluids.

4   If the temperature doesn't go down, sponge the child with lukewarm water for about 20 minutes. Don't immerse the child or infant in a tub—the temperature will go down more quickly if the wet skin is exposed to air currents.

5   Dry and dress the child in comfortable but not overly warm clothing. Monitor the child's temperature and repeat steps 3 to 5, as necessary, until medical help is reached.

6   If the child has a convulsion:

◆ don't restrain the child, but protect her from injury by removing hard objects and gently guiding movements

◆ loosen constrictive clothing

◆ when the convulsions stop, place the child into the best recovery position for their age.

Warning

◆ Do not give ASA (e.g. Aspirin®) to children or adolescents because it may cause Reye's syndrome, a life-threatening condition.

◆ Do not use cold water when sponging the child—this may cause more serious problems. Only use lukewarm water.

Bronchial asthma

Bronchial asthma (often called, simply, "asthma") is an illness in which the person has repeated attacks (asthmatic attacks) of shortness of breath. These usually include wheezing and coughing. Between attacks, the person has no trouble breathing. More children have asthma than adults. In half of these children, the condition goes away by the time they are adults.

Asthmatic attacks are often caused by certain common **triggers**, such as having a cold. Other common triggers are shown at the right. People with asthma can avoid the things that trigger an asthmatic attack, but even with this precaution, an asthmatic attack can occur unexpectedly.

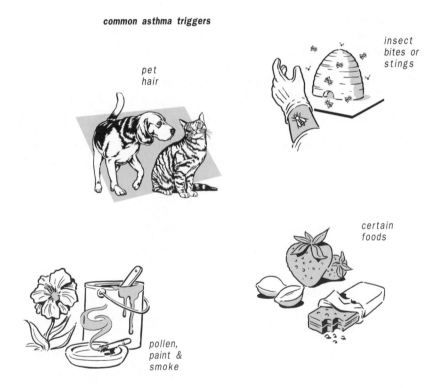

common asthma triggers

pet hair

insect bites or stings

certain foods

pollen, paint & smoke

In an asthmatic attack, air flow to the lungs is reduced. How much it is reduced determines whether the attack is mild or severe. A mild asthmatic attack can simply be annoying; a severe asthmatic attack can be fatal.

Signs and symptoms of a severe asthmatic attack

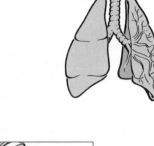

- ◆ shortness of breath with obvious trouble breathing

- ◆ coughing or wheezing (a whistling noise caused by air moving through narrowed airways)
  - may get louder or stop

- ◆ fast and shallow breathing

- ◆ casualty sitting upright trying to breathe

- ◆ bluish colour in the face (cyanosis)

- ◆ anxiety, tightness in the chest

- ◆ fast pulse rate, shock

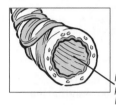

- ◆ restlessness at first, and then fatigue
  - the casualty becomes tired from trying so hard to breathe

healthy air passageway in the lungs

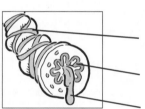

during an asthmatic attack, airflow in the lungs is reduced three ways:
- the muscles around the air passages tighten

- the inner linings of the air passages swell

- the amount and thickness of mucus increases

Asthma medications

There are a variety of asthma medications and the casualty may have more than one type.

First aid for an asthma attack

As a first aider, your help will only be needed when an asthmatic attack is severe. In a mild asthmatic attack, the casualty will be able to manage on her own.

To asssist a casualty suffering a severe asthma attack:

1 Begin ESM—do a scene survey and a primary survey. As soon as you identify a severe asthma attack, send for medical help.

2 Have the casualty stop any activity and place them in the most comfortable position for breathing. This is usually sitting upright with arms resting on a table.

3 Help the casualty take their prescribed medication.

4 Give ongoing casualty care. Stay with the casualty until medical help takes over. Give plenty of reassurance since fear and anxiety may cause the casualty to breathe faster, making the situation worse.

How to help a casualty take medication for a severe asthmatic attack

Often, a person with asthma carries medication in the form of a metered-dose inhaler (puffer). Usually the person can give himself this medication without help. But a person could need help during a severe asthmatic attack. A first aider can help a casualty to take his medication.

An inhaler delivers a premeasured amount of medication. For all medication to reach the lungs, it must be used properly. Always read and follow the manufacturer's instructions.

To help a casualty with asthma medication

1 Shake the container, then remove the cap.

2 Tell the casualty to breathe out completely in a relaxed manner. Then tell her to breathe in slowly and deeply—as they do, press the canister to release the medication. The cannister can be in the mouth or approx 4 finger-widths from the mouth.

3 Tell the casualty to hold their breath for 10 seconds so the medication can spread out in the lungs. Then tell them to breathe normally, so the medication won't be expelled. If more doses are needed, wait at least 30 seconds to one minute before repeating these steps.

Using a spacer (aero chamber)

When the medication comes out of the inhaler, it may be deposited on the back of the throat. To reduce this problem, use a spacer. It traps the particles of the spray, allowing the casualty to inhale more effectively.

spacer   inhaler

Small children and other casualties who have difficulty coordinating their inhaling with your releasing the medication, will find a spacer helpful. It allows them to inhale two or three times before the medication is completely dispelled. A mask can be attached to the device to make taking the medication easier.

 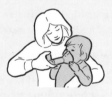

spacer with mask attached

If the casualty complains of throat irritation after using the inhaler, have them gargle or rinse their mouth with water.

If the casualty is unable to breathe in deeply before using the inhaler, using the spacer and having the casualty take three or four normal breaths from the spacer will help.

Severe allergic reaction

A life-threatening breathing emergency can result from a severe allergic reaction called **anaphylaxis** (an-a-fi-lak-sis). This reaction usually happens when a substance to which the casualty is very sensitive enters the body. Anaphylaxis can also be caused by exercise or have no cause. Anaphylaxis is a serious medical emergency that needs urgent medical attention.

Anaphylaxis can happen within seconds, minutes or hours of a substance entering the body. As a rule the sooner the casualty's body reacts, the worse the reaction will be.

Signs and symptoms of anaphylaxis	
The early signs and symptoms of anaphylaxis may include:	**As anaphylaxis progresses, the signs and symptoms may include:**
itchy, flushed skin, raised skin rash (hives)	pale skin and/or cyanosis
sneezing, running nose and watery eyes	anxiety and perhaps a severe headache
swelling of the airway	wheezing, chest feels like it's being squeezed
a "lump" or "tickle" in the throat that won't go away	breathing difficulties, coughing
coughing	pulse is rapid and irregular
sense of impending doom	shock, wrist pulse may be hard to find
nausea and vomiting	swelling of the lips, tongue, throat, hands and feet
	unconsciousness, stopped breathing, stopped heart (cardiac arrest)

First aid for a severe allergic reaction

1 Begin ESM—do a scene survey and a primary survey. As soon as you identify a severe allergic reaction, send for medical help.

2 Have the casualty stop any activity and place them in the most comfortable position for breathing. This is usually sitting upright with arms resting on a table.

3 Help the casualty take their prescribed medication. Some people with known allergies carry medication with them.

4 Give ongoing casualty care. Stay with the casualty until medical help takes over. Give plenty of reassurance since fear and anxiety may cause the casualty to breathe faster, making the situation worse.

How to help with medication for anaphylaxis

Anaphylaxis medication is injected into the body with a needle. The most popular product is explained here. These devices are designed for simple use and give the right amount of medication with each injection. If the casualty cannot give the injection to himself, you may have to do it.

EpiPen® Auto-Injector

The EpiPen® Auto-Injector is a disposable drug-delivery system with a spring-activated, concealed needle. An EpiPen® Auto-Injector delivers a single dose of medication. A casualty may have more than one auto-injector for multiple doses.

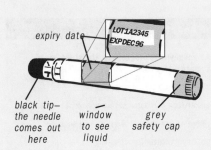

expiry date

LOT 1A2345
EXP DEC 96

black tip— the needle comes out here

window to see liquid

grey safety cap

To use the EpiPen® Auto-Injector

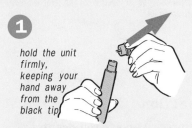

1

hold the unit firmly, keeping your hand away from the black tip

Take the unit out of the plastic case. Check the expiry date and pull off the grey safety cap—once this is off, any pressure on the black tip will activate the unit.

- ◆ If the liquid in the syringe is brown, do not use it. It should be clear and have no colour.
- ◆ If the device has expired (check the expiry date) do not use it.
- ◆ If you or anyone else is injected by mistake, get medical help.

2

only use the auto-injector on the fleshy part of the outer thigh

EpiPen® Auto-Injector can be given through lightweight clothing

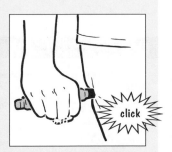

click

Firmly jab the black tip into the outer thigh until the unit activates—you'll feel and hear a "click." Hold the EpiPen® Auto-Injector in place for ten seconds, then pull it straight out.

3

After the injection, keep the casualty warm and avoid any exertion. If the casualty's condition doesn't get better in 10 minutes, give another dose if the casualty has one. The medication will begin to wear off within 10 to 20 minutes—get medical help right away.

What to do with the Auto-Injector

Bend the needle now coming out of the black tip of the unit against something—never touch it. Put the broken needle and the used unit back in the plastic case and take it to the hospital with the casualty.

Medical Conditions - Activity

· ·

· · · · · · · · · · **Diabetes** · · · · · · · · ·

1. In a healthy person, the body produces the _____ needed to allow cells to take up sugar and convert the sugar into energy.

2. _____ is a condition in which there is either not enough insulin in the blood or there is enough insulin but the cells cannot use the insulin properly.

3. Signs and symptoms of hypoglycemia include:

   a) _____   b) _____

   c) _____   d) _____.

4. Signs and symptoms of hyperglycemia include:

   a) _____   b) _____

   c) _____   d) _____.

5. The casualty may be wearing a _____ that will give you more information about their condition.

6. In the case of diabetic emergency, you should give the casualty _____ usually in the form of _____.

· · · · · · · · · · **Seizures** · · · · · · · · ·

7. A _____ is caused by abnormal electrical activity in the brain.

8. During a seizure you should:

   a) _____

   b) _____

   c) _____

   d) _____ .

9. After a seizure you should:

   a) _____

   b) _____ .

10. In the case of fever emergencies in children you should:

   a) _____

   b) _____ .

Medical Conditions - Activity

• •

· · · · · · · · · · Asthma · · · · · · · · ·

11. _____ is an illness in which the person has repeated attacks of shortness of breath.

12. Signs and symptoms of an asthmatic attack include:

   a) _____

   b) _____

   c) _____

   d) _____ .

13. Examples of triggers for an asthmatic attack include:

   a) _____   b) _____

   c) _____   d) _____ .

14. Often, a person with asthma carries medication referred to as a _____ . This device delivers a premeasured amount of medication.

· · · · · · · · · · Anaphylaxis · · · · · · · · ·

15. A life-threatening breathing emergency can result from a severe allergic reaction called _____ .

16. Signs and symptoms of the allergic reaction may include:

   a) _____

   b) _____

   c) _____

   d) _____ .

17. Anaphylaxis medication is injected into the body with a needle often by way of an _____ .

18. After using the medication, ensure the casualty gets _____ .

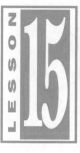

- Provide first aid for minor wounds

- Take measures to prevent further contamination and infection of minor wounds

- Describe minor wound complications

- Apply commercially prepared adhesive dressings and bandages

- Provide first aid for a casualty with a minor wound

- Provide first aid for a casualty with a second degree burn

- Complete first aid documentation

BC

Minor soft tissue wounds

1

Minor soft tissue wounds involve the skin and underlying soft tissue and do not present complications such as severe bleeding, excessive swelling, infection, nerve damage, circulation impairment or severe pain. Wounds with any of these serious complications require immediate medical attention.

Straight-edged laceration

Although most minor wounds can be adequately treated by the first aider alone, some minor wounds are slow to heal or prone to infection and should be referred to a medical doctor.

Minor wounds that should be referred to medical help:

- gaping wounds that are difficult to close

- deep wounds

- wounds over joints where underlying structures may be damaged

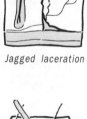

Jagged laceration

- wounds with embedded dirt or other foreign material

- human and animal bites

- significant second degree burns and all thrid degree burns

- facial wounds that maybe leave a visible scar

2

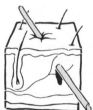

Puncture wound

Which of the following minor wounds should be referred to medical help? Indicate ✓ your choice in the squares provided.

- ☐ A. Split open wound to the palm of the hand that is difficult to close.
- ☐ B. Deep wound over a knuckle.
- ☐ C. Small cut in the surface of the skin.
- ☐ D. Wound caused by a rusty nail that is lodged in the tissue.

Open and closed wounds

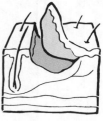

3

Minor soft tissue wounds may be **open** or **closed**. Blood loss from open wounds is minimal and bleeding is easily controlled. The aim of first aid for open wounds is to control bleeding and prevent infection.

Open wound

First aid for open wounds

▶ **control bleeding**

▶ **assess wound and surrounding area**

▶ **cleanse area around wound**

▶ **cleanse wound**

▶ **dress and bandage**

▶ **determine need for medical referral**

▶ **complete records**

In closed wounds the skin remains intact. Closed wounds result from impact with a blunt object or from excessive pressure or force. When a large amount of tissue is injured, swelling occurs. Excess swelling may compress major blood vessels and nerves and result in impaired circulation, loss of feeling, loss of ability to move the part, or increased pain.

Closed wounds that result in impaired circulation or nerve function require urgent medical attention.

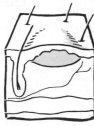

Closed Wound

FOR ALL MINOR WOUNDS -

Check circulation below the injury and compare it to the opposite limb by—

- comparing skin colour and temperature

- comparing the rate at which colour returns after pinching the nailbeds

Check nerve function below the injury and compare it to the opposite limb by—

- asking the person if they can move the part

- asking the person if they can feel it when you touch the part

First aid for closed wounds

▶ **examine injury and surrounding area**

▶ **determine need for medical attention**

▶ **bandage with light pressure to control swelling**

▶ **apply cold at 15 minute intervals for the first 48 hours**

4

From the options below, indicate ☑ the best completion to the following statement. The aim of first aid for open wounds is to:

❑ A.   Prevent swelling.

❑ B.   Refer the casualty to medical help.

❑ C.   Control bleeding and prevent infection.

❑ D.   Check the area around the wound.

Wound healing and infection

. . . .

5

As healing occurs, slight redness, swelling and tenderness will naturally appear around the edges of a wound. Excess redness, swelling and pain may, however, indicate infection.

Infection occurs when harmful bacteria grow within a wound. Signs of infection are not apparent immediately after injury and may take from one to several days to develop. Infection is recognized by the presence of:

- redness and/or red streaks extending away from the wound

- heat

- swelling

- local tenderness

- pus (an accumulation of dead tissue cells, white blood cells and bacteria)

Tetanus

Tetanus is a serious infectious disease caused by bacteria from animal faeces found in soil and dust. Tetanus may occur in any size or type of wound. Signs of tetanus, which include headache, fever, and muscle spasm may take several days to develop.

This life-threatening infection can be prevented if all wounds receive proper treatment and all patients with wounds have up-to-date immunization.

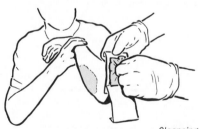 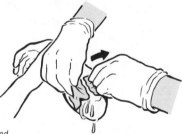

Cleansing of a wound

. . . .

6

Mark each of the following statements as either true (**T**) or false (**F**):

❑ A. Slight redness, swelling and tenderness always indicate infection.

❑ B. All infected wounds should be referred to medical help.

❑ C. Tetanus is a serious infection.

❑ D. There are no precautions against the occurrence of tetanus.

To reduce the risk of infection

7

All wounds are contaminated to some degree. From the moment of injury, there is the risk of infection that continues until the wound is completely healed. Although controlling bleeding is the priority, first aiders should use the cleanest materials available to cover the wound.

Follow these principles when cleaning a minor wound.

- ◆ cleanse all minor wounds prior to bandaging

- ◆ wash your hands before and after handling wounds in addition to wearing gloves

wash your hands with s and w

- ◆ re-examine wounds for signs of infection after the first 24-48 hours and periodically thereafter until the wound is completely healed

- ◆ ensure the casualty has been immunized for tetanus within the past five years

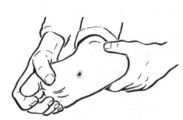

superficial puncture wound

Cleanse the wound thoroughly and soak in a soap solution for 15-20 minutes

Continue soaks 3-4 times a day for 48 hours

8

Which of the following actions are good first aid procedures to prevent further contamination and infection? Check ☑ the correct answers.

- ❑ A. Blow loose dirt away from the wound.

- ❑ B. Clean small wounds before applying a dressing.

- ❑ C. Wipe away from the wound with a clean piece of gauze to remove dirt.

- ❑ D. Once covered, don't remove the bandage until the wound is completely healed.

Dressings and bandages

· ·

9

Dressings and bandages are the basic tools of first aid. The type of dressing and bandage and the techniques for applying them will vary according to the type of injury.

- **Sterile dressings**
  Sterile dressings provide the initial covering for open wounds.

- **Soaker or drainage dressings**
  Drainage dressings are placed on top of sterile dressings and act as a sponge to soak up excess fluid.

- **Bandages**
  Bandages hold dressings in place and maintain pressure to control bleeding and prevent swelling.

General rules for applying dressings and bandages

- avoid touching any part of a dressing that will contact the wound

- never talk or cough over a wound or dressing

- use sufficient dressings to extend beyond the edges of the wound

- apply bandages firmly enough to hold dressings in place and control bleeding, but not so tight that they impair circulation

- make sure the bandage covers all the dressings underneath

- when possible, leave fingernails or toenails exposed to check circulation

- check circulation and nerve function before and after bandaging

- ensure the bandage is large enough to cover all of the dressings.

· ·

10

Check ✓ the correct completions of the following statement. Circulation and nerve function checks should be performed:

- ❑ A. Before and after bandaging a wound to a limb

- ❑ B. By a medical doctor only

- ❑ C. For all major and minor wounds to limbs

- ❑ D. For major wounds only

Dressings and bandages

11

Wound closures

Wound closures are special adhesive strips used to bring wound edges together to assist healing. For small gaping wounds without complications, wound closures eliminate the need for stitches. Do not apply wound closures if you are referring the casualty to medical aid.

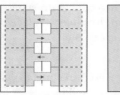

Butterfly closures   Transparent strip closures

Commercially prepared adhesive dressings

Commercially prepared adhesive dressings combine the dressing, padding and bandage all in one and are available in a variety of shapes and sizes.

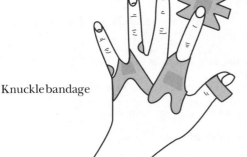

Fingertip bandage

Strip bandage

Knuckle bandage

Knuckle bandage

12 Choose ☑ the best answer from either choice 1 or choice 2:

Choice 1

- ❑ A. A knuckle bandage is used to bring the edges of a gaping wound together to assist healing.

- ❑ B. A strip bandage is a type of adhesive dressing you can buy.

Choice 2

- ❑ A. A butterfly closure is used to bring the edge of a gaping wound together to assist healing.

- ❑ B. A fingertip bandage is placed on a wound at the base of the finger.

Burns

13

Heat is the most common cause of burns. Other causes include contact with corrosive chemicals, electrical currents and over-exposure to radiation.

First degree (*surface*) burns

A first degree burn affects only the outer layers of the skin and results in redness, swelling and tenderness. This type of burn usually heals well. First degree burns covering an area larger than the size of the casualty's hand should receive medical attention.

Second and third degree (*deep*) burns

Second degree burns involve the formation of blisters, which may be intact or broken, with an area of surrounding redness. Significant second degree burns (such as burns to the face or hands) should be referred to a medical doctor. Third degree burns destroy the skin and affect deeper structures. These burns must always be referred to medical help.

First aid for burns

• cool the burn

• assess the degree of damage

• cover with a clean dressing

• bandage lightly

• refer first and second degree burns to medical aid if the burn is larger than the size of the casualty's hand

• refer all significant second degree burns to areas such as the hands or face to medicl aid

• refer all third degree burns to medical aid

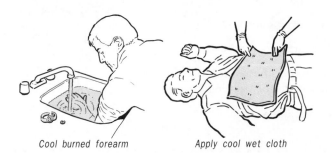

Cool burned forearm   Apply cool wet cloth

14

Mark each of the following statements as true (**T**) or false (**F**):

❑ A. All burns require medical attention.

❑ B. All deep burns require medical attention.

❑ C. Surface burns sometimes require medical attention.

❑ D. First degree burns involve the deep layers of the skin.

Eye injuries

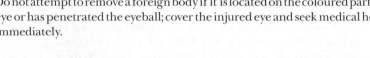

15

All eye injuries are potentially serious. Knowledge of the mechanism of injury (what happened) and the nature of the foreign material will enable you to provide appropriate first aid care. Particles of dust, grit or loose eyelashes are the most common foreign bodies found in eyes. In most cases these are easily removed.

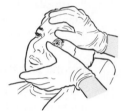

Do not attempt to remove a foreign body if it is located on the coloured part of the eye or has penetrated the eyeball; cover the injured eye and seek medical help immediately.

To remove loose foreign material from the eye:

Eye wash pitcher

♦ determine the history (what happened)

♦ determine the mechanism of injury

♦ wash hands and apply gloves

♦ clean around the eye

♦ flush the eye with water

Examination of the eye

♦ pull the upper lid over lower lashes

♦ inspect the lower eye and inside lid

♦ inspect the upper eye and inside lid

♦ examine the surface of the eye

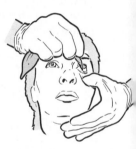

♦ remove the object with a moistened cotton-tipped applicator or corner of a sterile gauze pad

Eye wash with bottle

♦ complete a first aid record

Removal of loose material

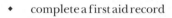

16

Mark each of the following completions to the statements below as true (**T**) or false (**F**).

A first aider may attempt to remove a loose foreign object from the eye, when the object is located on the:

❑ A. White part of the eye.

❑ B. Coloured part of the eye.

❑ C. Inside of the lower eyelid.

❑ D. Inside of the upper eyelid.

Documentation

• •

17

First aid record

All injuries, regardless how minor, must be recorded. First aid records must be kept at the workplace for at least 3 years. A sample first aid record is shown on page 15-10.

Blank copies of the first aid record form should be kept in the first aid kit, ready for use. Completed first aid records contain confidential information, and should be filed in a secure location.

WorkSafe BC Form 7A

If a worker is referred to a medical doctor or is advised to seek medical attention, the first aider must complete a WorkSafe BC Form 7A. A sample of the WorkSafe BC Form 7A is shown on page 15-11 and 15-12.

• •

18

Mark each of the following statements as either true (**T**) or false (**F**):

❑ A. A first aid record is a legal document.

❑ B. A first aid record is only required when the worker is sent to see a medical doctor

❑ C. A first aid record is always required.

❑ D. A WorkSafe BC First Aid Report (Form 7A) is required when a worker is referred to a medical doctor for a work release injury or illness.

FIRST AID RECORD

Sequence number _____

Date of injury or illness	Time of injury or illness
Name	Time and date reported
Occupation	

Description of Injury or Report of Illness (what happened)

Nature of Injury or Illness (signs and symptoms)

Treatment(s)

First aid attendant's signature	First aid attendant's name *(please print)*
Patient's signature	

Name of witnesses

1. _____

2. _____

3. _____

Referral of Case and Remarks (return to work/medical aid/ambulance)

55B23 (R01/06)

WORKERS' COMPENSATION BOARD OF BC

FIRST AID REPORT

Please answer all questions and complete this report in ink.

Supplementary to Employer's Form 7 "Employer's Report of Injury or Occupational Disease."

The following questions to be completed in full by First Aid Attendant, or other person rendering first aid. Please sign and attach to the Form 7 for submission to the address or fax number on page 2.

7A

WORKER'S LAST NAME *(please print)*		EMPLOYER'S NAME *(as registered with the Board)*	
Mr. Ms. Mrs. Miss			
First name(s)	Middle initial	Mailing address	
Mailing address		City	Postal code
City	Postal code	Location of plant or project where injury occurred	Postal code
Telephone number / Social insurance number / Date of birth (Month Day Year)		Type of business	Employer's telephone number
Weight (Feet Inches) / Height / Marital status ☐ Married ☐ Single ☐ Other		Worker's occupation	Worker's personal health number from BC CareCard

1. Date and time of injury _____ *(Month)* _____ *(Day)* 20 ___ , at ___ a.m. / p.m.

2. (a) Time of reporting to First Aid Attendant _____ *(Month)* _____ *(Day)* 20 ___ , at ___ a.m. / p.m.

   (b) How did the worker get to the First Aid Room? *(walk, stretcher, truck, etc.)* _____

   (c) By whom was the injured worker brought to the First Aid Room? _____

   (d) Was the worker unconscious following injury or exposure? ☐ Yes ☐ No   If yes, for how long? _____

   Was this based on personal observation? ☐ Yes ☐ No

3. (a) Please describe injuries found _____

   (b) Please give nature of initial first aid rendered _____

   (c) Please give dates and nature of subsequent treatments _____

4. When did the worker leave to see a physician or qualified practitioner? _____ *(Month)* _____ *(Day)* 20 ___ , at ___ a.m. / p.m.

   Did worker report to a physician or qualified practitioner as soon as advised? ☐ Yes ☐ No

5. Location and approximate distance to nearest physician or qualified practitioner

6. Please give name and address of physician or qualified practitioner

7. By what means was the worker transported to a physician or qualified practitioner?

First aid attendant's signature		Date
First aid certificate *(if any)* dated	Certificate number	Grade
Worker's statement of injury		

☞ **ADDITIONAL INFORMATION CAN BE RECORDED ON THE REVERSE SIDE OF THIS REPORT.**
Please see the reverse side of this report for telephone and fax numbers.

7A (R07/04) 1 of 2

Worker's last name	First name	Middle initial	Social insurance number	Claim number

Worker's personal health number from BC CareCard

Additional information

Mailing address for report and all claims correspondence: Workers' Compensation Board of BC
PO Box 8940 Stn Terminal
Vancouver BC V6B 1H9

Fax number: Local 604 233-9722 or toll free within BC 1 888 922-8803.

For additional information on the Workers' Compensation Board, please refer to our web site at **www.WorkSafebc.com**.

Telephone information

Call Centre: 604 231-8888 or toll free within BC 1 888 967-5377.

Occupational Disease Services: 604 276-3007 or toll free within BC 1 888 967-5377 (extension 3007).

 7A (R07/04) 2 of 2

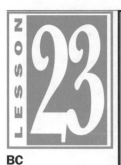

Objectives

- Apply basic knowledge of the respiratory system
- Perform mouth to mask artificial respiration (AR) on an adult casualty
- Perform mouth to mask (AR) on an adult casualty with suspected head/spinal injuries
- Determine ineffective breathing
- Perform assisted breathing

BC

Breathing emergencies

Continuous, effective breathing is vital for life. When a person's breathing is affected through injury or illness, their life can be in immediate danger. As a first aider, you have to be able to recognize a breathing emergency very quickly and know what first aid to give—the casualty's life may depend on it.

Hypoxia

A breathing emergency causes a lack of oxygen in the blood. This condition, called **hypoxia** can damage vital tissues and eventually cause death if not corrected. The causes of hypoxia are grouped under three headings:

- **lack of oxygen**—for example:

  - an environment where the oxygen level is low, such as at a high altitude

  - the oxygen is displaced by other gases, such as carbon monoxide, silo gas on a farm or hydrogen sulphide (H_2S) in an industrial setting

  - the oxygen in a small space is used up—for instance, a young child trapped in an old refrigerator quickly uses up all the air

- **blocked airway**—for example:

  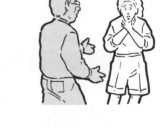

  - the casualty chokes on a foreign object, like food

  - the casualty is face up while unconscious and the tongue blocks the airway

  - the casualty's airway is swollen from an infection

- **ineffective breathing**—for example:

  - severe chest injury

  - inhalation injury (smoke inhalation)

    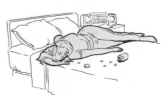

  - drug overdose

  - spinal cord injury

Artificial Respiration and Assisted Breathing

◆ **abnormal heart function**—the heart is not working properly, for example:

- an illness such as chronic obstructive pulmonary disease, pneumonia or congestive heart failure

- an injury to the head, spine, chest, etc.

- a drug overdose or poisoning

Requirements for effective breathing

To breathe effectively, we need at least the following:

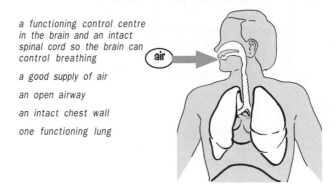

a functioning control centre in the brain and an intact spinal cord so the brain can control breathing

a good supply of air

an open airway

an intact chest wall

one functioning lung

Signs of normal, effective breathing

The most important signs the first aider uses to assess breathing are rate, rhythm and depth.

Breathing **rate** is the number of breaths (inhalations and exhalations) in one minute. The table below gives the range of normal breathing rates for adults. The table also gives the rates that are too slow and too fast. A breathing rate that is too slow or too fast is a sign of a breathing emergency.

Breathing rate – breaths per minute			
	range of normal rates	too slow	too fast
adult (over 8 years of age)	10 to 20	below 10	above 30

Breathing **rhythm** refers to the interval between breaths. In normal breathing, the intervals are even and breathing is effortless—this is regular breathing. In irregular breathing, the intervals between breaths are uneven. This usually indicates a respiratory disorder or distress.

Breathing **depth** refers to the amount of air moved in and out of the lungs with each breath. Learn to recognize the difference between normal breathing depth and shallow or deep breathing.

Other signs of normal breathing include:

- quiet and effortless breathing
- chest movement that is equal on both sides
- the person is alert and relaxed
- normal skin colour
- able to speak without taking a breath every few words

Signs of ineffective breathing

When a person is breathing normally, breathing is **effective**. This means the body is getting the oxygen it needs to function. As a person's breathing becomes more and more impaired, there is a point where the body needs more oxygen than it is getting. At this point, breathing becomes **ineffective**. There are different levels of ineffective breathing, as the illustration below shows. As a first aider, you need to be able to tell the difference between breathing that is "just a little" ineffective, where the casualty's life is not in immediate danger, and breathing that is very ineffective, where the casualty's life is in immediate danger. When breathing is very ineffective, the casualty has **severe breathing difficulties**.

Signs and symptoms of severe breathing difficulties

Look for the signs and symptoms below. Notice whether the person's condition changes over time. For example, if a person with breathing difficulties who was fully conscious begins to get drowsy, you know the breathing difficulties are severe and medical help is urgently needed.

person may be anxious, afraid, terrified, etc. because of the breathing difficulty (**dyspnea**)

breathing is difficult—the casualty is struggling for breath or gasping for air

breathing rate may be too fast or too slow

breathing rhythm may be irregular

breathing depth may be too shallow or too deep

breathing may be noisy or raspy

person may say he's "getting tired" from trying to breathe

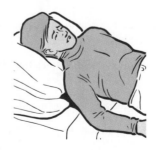

the casualty may be sweaty from working so hard at breathing

decreased level of consciousness

the lips, ears and fingernail beds look bluish (this bluish tinge is called **cyanosis**)

chest movement may be abnormal—the chest goes in and the abdomen puffs out during inhalation

there may be little or no chest movement or breathing effort

you may not be able to feel air moving in and out of the nose and mouth

First aid for stopped breathing – Artificial respiration (AR)

The vital organs of the body such as the brain and heart need a continuous supply of oxygen to stay alive. Artificial respiration (AR) is a way you can supply air to the lungs of a casualty who is not breathing.

In the second step of the primary survey, you check for breathing. If there is no breathing, you start AR, if trained to do so.

As you breathe, the air you exhale contains enough oxygen to keep a non-breathing person alive. Artificial respiration involves blowing this air into the casualty's lungs to deliver oxygen to the non-breathing person. The number of times you blow in one minute is called the **rate**—AR has to be given at the proper rate to make sure the casualty is getting enough oxygen.

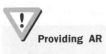

Providing AR

In order to know whether a casualty needs AR only (and not CPR) you need to know how to take a pulse. Because this is often difficult to accurately determine, artificial respiration is taught to health care providers and certain first responders only. Lay rescuers are no longer taught this skill.

There are a number of different techniques of AR and the one you use depends on the situation. These are:

- ◆ **mouth-to-mouth AR**—this is the most commonly used method of AR. The first aider pinches the casualty's nose closed and blows into their mouth

- ◆ **mouth-to-nose AR**—this method is used in situations where mouth-to-mouth is not appropriate, such as when your mouth won't cover the casualty's mouth. You hold the casualty's mouth closed and blow into his nose.

- ◆ **mouth-to-stoma AR**—this technique is for a casualty who has previously had a laryngectomy and breathes through a hole in their neck (called a stoma)

Artificial respiration can be given in a wide range of situations. In an emergency situation, keep the following in mind:

- ◆ you can start AR right away in any position (but it is best if the casualty is on their back on a firm, flat surface)

- ◆ you can continue AR while the casualty is being moved to safety by other rescuers

- ◆ you can give AR for a long time without getting too tired

Giving AR in some situations, may be more difficult than in others. When this happens, you have to do the best you can (based on your level of training) without putting yourself into danger. Sample situations are:

◆ when severe deforming injuries to the mouth and nose prevent a good seal around the mouth

◆ blood and/or other body fluids drain into the throat and block the airway when you try AR (do your best to drain the mouth)

◆ the casualty was poisoned by a toxic gas like hydrogen sulphide and coming in contact with the casualty may result in you being poisoned

◆ the casualty has a corrosive poison on the face or in the mouth, and you don't have a face mask

How to give artificial respiration

The following pages illustrate, in detail, how to give artificial respiration to adult casualties. The method is presented as a rescue sequence and shows all the actions you should take when you find an unresponsive casualty. These sequence follows the same steps as the scene survey and primary survey described in chapter 1, but here the casualty is given first aid for stopped breathing.

If there is breathing, assess whether the casualty is having severe breathing difficulties. If so, give first aid to make breathing more effective. If there are still severe breathing difficulties, assist breathing using the techniques of AR.

How to give assisted breathing

Assisted breathing helps a casualty with severe breathing difficulties to breathe more effectively. It is most useful when the casualty shows very little or no breathing effort. If breathing effort is good, the casualty will likely breathe better on his own. Start assisted breathing when you recognize the signs of severe breathing difficulties (see page 23-3).

The technique for assisted breathing is the same as for artificial respiration except for the timing of the ventilations. You seal your mouth around the casualty's mouth and/or nose and blow air into the lungs (use a face mask or shield if you have one). If the casualty is breathing too slowly, give a breath each time the casualty inhales,

plus an extra breath in between the casualty's own breaths. Give one breath every five or six seconds for a total of 10-12 breaths per minute for an adult casualty.

If the casualty is breathing too fast, give one breath on every second inhalation by the casualty. This will hopefully slow down the casualty's own breathing. Give a total of 10-12 breaths per minute.

If the casualty is conscious, explain what you are going to do and why. Reassure the casualty often and encourage him to try to breathe at a good rate with good depth. If the casualty doesn't want you to assist their breathing, explain why it is important. If the casualty still doesn't want you to assist his breathing, don't.

Mouth-to-mouth artificial respiration – adult casualty

You arrive at a scene...an unconscious adult (someone over 8 years of age) is lying on the floor.

1 Begin ESM—start the scene survey.

- -

2 Assess responsiveness. If there is no response, go to step 3.

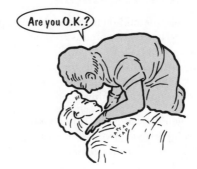

ask the casualty if they are O.K. Assess any response.

gently tap the shoulders

- -

3 Send or go for medical help an an AED if available.

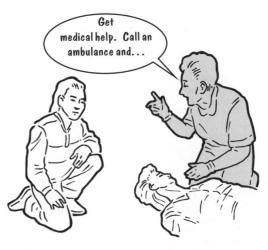

If you are alone, it may be best for you to go for medical help—see page 1-9.

4 Place the casualty face up, protecting the head and neck during any movement. Open the airway by tilting the head.

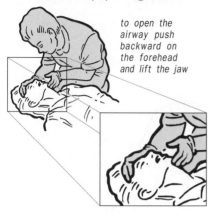

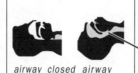

to open the airway push backward on the forehead and lift the jaw

airway closed   airway open

when the head is tilted back, the tongue is lifted off the back of the throat, opening the airway

5 Check for normal breathing for up to 10 seconds.

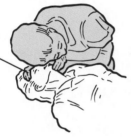

keep the head tilted

place your ear just above the casualty's nose and mouth

look. . . for chest movement

listen. . . for sounds of breathing

feel. . . for breath on your cheek

Agonal Breathing

Agonal breathing may be present in cardiac arrest casualties. Casualties will have gasping with no regular pattern or depth. Do not confuse this with regular breathing.

If there is no breathing, go to step 6.

6 Breathe into the casualty twice. For an adult casualty, blow for 1 second. Use enough air to make the chest rise.

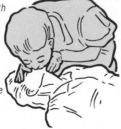

take a normal breath and seal your mouth around the casualty's mouth

pinch the nostrils

blow in and watch for the chest to rise

move your mouth away and release the nostrils to allow the air to escape

look for the chest to fall, listen for air sounds and feel for air being exhaled against your cheek

give another breath and go to step 7

If the chest doesn't rise when you blow:

♦ reopen the airway by tilting the head

♦ pinch the nose again

♦ make a better seal around the mouth

♦ try blowing again

If the chest still doesn't rise, give first aid for choking—see page 3-7, step 7.

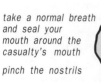

7   Check for a pulse at the neck. There is a carotid pulse on either side of the neck—feel for a pulse on the side closest to you—**do not feel or compress both sides at the same time**

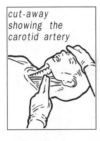

cut-away showing the carotid artery

First aider's view of the pulse check

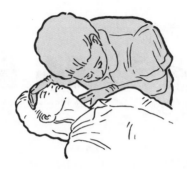

keep the head tilted

slide 2 fingers into the groove of the neck just down from the Adam's apple

press gently to detect the pulse, take no longer than 10 seconds

Be aware that pulses can be hard to find. If there is no pulse or if you are not sure, do not delay, start CPR and apply an AED—

If there is a pulse, continue AR—see step 8, below.

- -

8   Breathe into the casualty once every five to six seconds (10 to 12 times a minute). After one minute of AR, recheck for a pulse for no more than 10 seconds, and at the same time, look, listen and feel for breathing:

    ◆ if there is no pulse start CPR and apply AED

    ◆ if there is a pulse and breathing, continue the primary survey—see page 1-13

Don't blow too hard

If you blow into a casualty too hard or faster than the recommended rate the air may go into the stomach instead of the lungs. This can cause a few problems. Only blow hard enough to make the chest rise.

    ◆ if there is a pulse and still no breathing, continue AR. Recheck for a pulse every few minutes. Keep giving AR until the casualty starts to breathe on their own, medical help takes over or you are too tired to continue

How to give AR when you suspect a head or spinal injury

Note that this technique is only intended for health care providers and first responders

The usual AR technique involves moving the head and neck to open the airway. If the casualty has a head or neck injury, this movement could cause paralysis or even death.

When you suspect a head or spinal injury, prevent head and neck movement and open the airway using the **jaw-thrust without head-tilt** as shown below.

1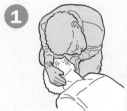

place your hands on either side of the casualty's head so the head and neck cannot move

Tell the casualty not to move. Support the head and neck and assess responsiveness. Send for medical help if the casualty is unresponsive.

2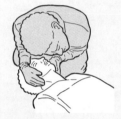

Check for breathing in the position found. Look, listen and feel for signs of breathing.

3

open the airway—press on the chin to open the mouth and lift the jaw

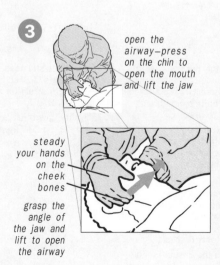

steady your hands on the cheek bones

grasp the angle of the jaw and lift to open the airway

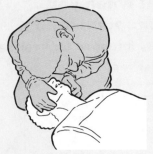

look. . . for chest movement

listen. . . for sounds of breathing

feel. . . for breath on your cheek

If you must reposition the casualty to properly assess him or give AR, move or turn him as a unit as much as possible.

Check for signs of breathing for up to 10 seconds while holding the airway open with the jaw thrust.

5

push your cheek against the nose to seal the nose

keep lifting the jaw to hold the airway open

take a normalbreath and blow slowly for 1 second and watch for the chest to rise

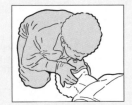

Ventilating a casualty using the jaw-thrust without head-tilt and a face mask (pocket mask)

If there is no breathing, put your mouth over the casualty's mouth and press your cheek against the casualty's nose to seal it. Blow into the casualty's mouth and watch for the chest to rise.

If the chest rises, give another breath and continue AR. If the chest doesn't rise, try opening the airway again with the jaw thrust, but this time:

◆ tilt the head slightly backwards—just enough to open the airway (although these actions move the neck, it is more important to get air into the casualty's lungs than to protect the neck)

◆ try to breathe into the casualty again.

If the chest still does not rise, conclude the airway is blocked by a foreign object and start first aid for choking—see page 3-7, step 7.

Using the jaw thrust, continue giving AR as described on 23-7, step 6.

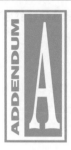

Emergency scene management—
Unresponsive casualty

ADDENDUM A

An unconscious adult casualty is lying face up. The first aider witnessed the casualty's collapse. There is a bystander nearby.

Activity

SCENE SURVEY

- take charge of the situation

- call out for help and assess hazards at the scene

- determine the number of casualties, what happened, and the mechanism of injury

- identify yourself and offer to help

- assess responsiveness

- send for medical help

Performance Guidelines

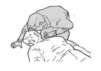

Approach from within the casualty's line of sight

Ask bystanders to standby. Make the area safe. To protect yourself, put on non- latex or vinyl gloves if available

Since you witnessed the incident, you know what happened and the mechanism of injury *[You do not suspect head or spinal injuries]*

Identify yourself and ask for consent. If the casualty doesn't respond, you have implied consent

Ask, "Are you O.K.?" and gently tap the casualty's shoulders
[Casualty does not respond]

Give the following information: what happened, location, and that the casualty is unresponsive

PRIMARY SURVEY (ABCs)

- airway

- breathing

- circulation

A Open the airway using the head-tilt, chin-lift

B Look, listen and feel for up to 10 seconds to check for breathing   *[Casualty is breathing]*

Assess the quality and the rate of breathing by placing a hand on the casualty's chest
[Breathing is quiet, occurs without effort and with an even, steady rhythm]

C Check radial pulse and skin
[Pulse is present; Skin is pale, warm and dry]

Check for hidden, severe, external bleeding and signs of internal bleeding using the rapid body survey *[Casualty has no apparent bleeding or deformities]*

Activity

SECONDARY SURVEY

Performance Guidelines

[Secondary survey is not required as medical help will arrive soon]

ONGOING CASUALTY CARE

- monitor casualty's condition

- record the events

- report on what happened

Reassure the casualty and loosen tight clothing at the neck, chest and waist.

Place the casualty into the **recovery position.**
If possible, place a blanket underneath the casualty before turning.

Cover the casualty, do not give anything by mouth. Protect the casualty's belongings

Reassess ABCs

Take notes of the casualty's condition and any changes that may occur

Tell medical attendants what happened. *[Casualty remains unconscious]*

Emergency scene management—Responsive casualty

An adult casualty has fallen and hit her head, and is lying face up. The casualty can speak clearly and open her eyes when spoken to. Two bystanders are present who witnessed the incident.

Activity	Performance Guidelines

SCENE SURVEY

- take charge of the situation

Approach from within the casualty's line of sight. Tell the casualty not to move

- call out for help

Ask bystanders to standby

- assess hazards at the scene

Make the area safe. To protect yourself, put on non- latex or vinyl gloves if available

- determine the number of casualties, what happened, and the mechanism of injury

Question the casualty to determine what happened and the mechanism of injury *[Head/spinal injuries are suspected]*

- identify yourself and offer to help
- send for medical help

Identify yourself and ask for consent

Give the following information: what happened, location, and the condition of the casualty

- assess responsiveness

Provide support for the casualty's head and neck since head/spinal injuries are suspected—ask, "Are you OK?"

PRIMARY SURVEY (ABCs)

*[A conscious casualty **is** responsive]*

- airway

A   Ask the casualty, "Where are you hurt?" *[The casualty can speak clearly therefore has a clear airway]*

Instruct a bystander to steady and support the casualty's head and neck

- breathing

B   Check for effectiveness of breathing. Ask, "How is your breathing?" [*The casualty moans.*] Place a hand on the casualty's chest and count the number of breaths per minute [*Breathing is effective*]

- circulation

C   Check the radial pulse and the skin [*the pulse is present; skin is pale, warm and dry*]

Check for hidden, severe, external bleeding and signs of internal bleeding with the rapid body survey [*Casualty has no apparent bleeding or deformities*]

Emergency scene management—Responsive casualty - Cont'd...

Activity

Performance Guidelines

[Secondary survey is not required as medical help will arrive soon]

SECONDARY SURVEY

Continue support for the head and neck and do not move the casualty

ONGOING CASUALTY CARE

Reassure the casualty and loosen tight clothing at the neck, chest and waist. Cover the casualty. Do not give anything by mouth

Recheck ABCs often

- monitor casualty's condition

Take notes of the casualty's condition and any changes that may occur—protect the casualty's belongings

- record the events

- report on what happened

Tell medical attendants what happened, the casualty's condition and what first aid was given *[Casualty remains conscious]*

Choking–Adult conscious becoming unconscious

An adult casualty is grasping at her throat and coughing forcefully. A bystander is present.

Activity	Performance Guidelines

Activity

SCENE SURVEY

- take charge of the situation
- call out for help and assess hazards at the scene
- determine the number of casualties, what happened, and the mechanism of injury
- identify yourself and offer to help

PRIMARY SURVEY (ABCs)

- airway

- send for medical help

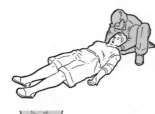

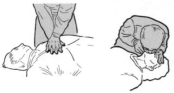

Performance Guidelines

Approach from within the casualty's line of sight

Ask the bystander to stand by. Make the area safe. To protect yourself, put on non- latex or vinyl gloves if available

Ask "Are you choking?" [The casualty is coughing forcefully]

Identify yourself and ask for consent. If the casualty doesn't respond, you have implied consent

A   Do not intervene at this time— encourage coughing

Watch for signs of complete obstruction

[The casualty now cannot cough, breathe or speak]

When coughing stops:

Stand behind the casualty and landmark—give inward and upward abdominal thrusts until the airway is cleared or the casualty becomes unconscious

[The casualty becomes unconscious]
Ease the casualty to the floor on her back

Give the following information: what happened, location, and that the casualty is choking and unconscious

Look in the mouth [Nothing is visible]

Open the airway and check for breathing [No breathing]

Try to ventilate [Chest does not rise]

Reposition the head, check the seals and try to ventilate again [Chest still does not rise]

Give 30 chest compressions. Repeat looking in the mouth, attempts to ventilate and chest compressions until the airway is cleared, medical help takes over or you cannot continue any longer [The object is seen and removed]

Choking–Adult conscious becoming unconscious - Cont'd

Activity

- breathing
- circulation

Complete the primary survey

SECONDARY SURVEY

ONGOING CASUALTY CARE

Performance Guidelines

B   Give 1 breath checking that the chest rises and falls *[Chest rises and falls.]* Give a second breath, watching the chest rise and fall. Assess rate and quality of breathing by placing hand on casualty's chest *[Breathing is effective]*

C   Circulation- Check for shock- *skin is cold and clammy]*

[Secondary survey is not required as medical help will arrive soon]

Give first aid for shock, monitor casualty's condition. Continue to check ABCs until medical help takes over. Record the events along with any changes that may occur and report to medical attendants when they arrive

Choking–Adult (pregnant or larger than rescuer)

A woman in an advanced stage of pregnancy appears to be choking and she cannot cough, breathe or speak.   A bystander is present.

Activity	Performance Guidelines

SCENE SURVEY

- take charge of the situation
- call out for help and assess hazards at the scene
- determine the number of casualties, what happened, and the mechanism of injury
- identify yourself and offer to help

PRIMARY SURVEY (ABCs)

- airway

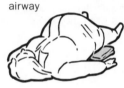

- send for medical help

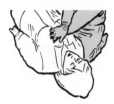

- breathing

Approach from within the casualty's line of sight

Ask the bystander to stand by. Make the area safe. To protect yourself, put on latex or vinyl gloves if available

Ask "Are you choking?" *[The casualty cannot cough, breathe or speak]*

You have identified yourself and asked for consent. If the casualty doesn't respond, you have implied consent

A   Identify the degree of obstruction

Stand behind the casualty and landmark—give inward **chest** thrusts until the airway is cleared or the casualty becomes unconscious

[The casualty becomes unconscious]
Ease the casualty to the floor on her back. Place a wedge under her right hip, if readily available

Give the following information: what happened, location, the number of casualties and that the casualty is choking, and unconscious

Look in the mouth *[Nothing is visible]*

Open the airway and check for breathing *[No breathing]*

Try to ventilate *[Chest does not rise]*

Reposition the head, check the seals and try to ventilate again   *[Chest still does not rise]*

Landmark - Give 30 chest compressions—repeat looking in the mouth, attempts to ventilate and chest compressions until the airway is cleared, medical help takes over or you cannot continue any longer *[The object is seen and removed]*

B   Give 1 breath checking that the chest rises and falls. *[Chest rises and falls]* Give a second breath, watching the chest rise and fall

Activity	Performance Guidelines
	[The casualty is breathing, but remains unconscious] Assess the quality and rate of breathing by placing a hand on the casualty's chest. *Breathing is effective*
• circulation	C Circulation- Check signs of shock (skin temperature and condition), *[skin is cold and clammy]*
Complete the primary survey	
SECONDARY SURVEY	*[Secondary survey is not required as medical help will arrive soon]*
ONGOING CASUALTY CARE	Give first aid for shock, monitor casualty's condition. Continue to check ABCs until medical help takes over. Record the events, with any changes that may occur and report to medical attendants when they arrive

One rescuer CPR–Adult

An adult casualty is lying face up. There are no bystanders. The first aider witnessed the incident. There is a telephone nearby.

Activity

Performance Guidelines

SCENE SURVEY

- take charge of the situation
- call out for help and assess hazards at the scene
- determine the number of casualties, what happened, and the mechanism of injury
- identify yourself and offer to help

- assess responsiveness

- send/call for medical help and get AED

Approach from within the casualty's line of sight

Make the area safe. To protect yourself, put on non- latex or vinyl gloves if available

You witnessed the collapse and you do not suspect head or spinal injuries

Identify yourself and ask for consent. If the casualty doesn't respond, you have implied consent

Ask, "Are you O.K.?" and gently tap the casualty's shoulders
[Casualty does not respond]

Give the following information: what happened, location, and that the casualty is unresponsive

PRIMARY SURVEY (ABCs)

- airway
- breathing

- circulation

A Open the airway using the head-tilt, chin-lift

B Look, listen and feel for up to 10 seconds to check for breathing *[Casualty is not breathing]* Give two breaths (1 second each) watching the chest to make sure it rises and falls *[The chest rises and falls]*

C *Check carotid pulse for up to 10 seconds. If no pulse, being CPR*

Give cycles of 30 compressions and 2 ventilations

Continue CPR until the circulation is restored, until medical help takes over, until another first aider trained in CPR takes over or until you are physically exhausted and unable to continue *[The casualty has no signs of life]*

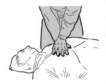

SECONDARY SURVEY

ONGOING CASUALTY CARE

In this situation the first aider continues CPR until medical help arrives. The first aider has not progressed from the primary survey *before help arrives*

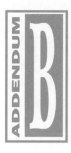
ADDENDUM B

Wound Care Handouts

Small Wounds and Cuts

You have an open wound.

With proper care it should start to feel better in about 3-4 days.

The healing process will be more effective by following this advice:

- Keep dressing clean and dry
- If skin closures have been applied, they are to remain in place for 7-10 days
- When bathing or showering, cover dressings to prevent moisture from entering
- You should notice some redness around the wound, which is the natural healing process
- You may also notice slight pain the day following the injury, this is also part of the natural healing process
- Report to first aid within 24-48 hours after the injury
- The first aid attendant will reassess and re-bandage the wound

If at any time you notice that pain, redness, and swelling increase significantly or if you see pus or red streaks, report to the first aid attendant, who may refer you to medical aid. If the condition becomes significantly worse while you're not at work and you decide to seek medical aid, notify the attendant as soon as possible.

Soft Tissue Injury at a Joint (possible ankle sprain)

A sprain is a stretching, or a partial or complete tearing of a ligament at a joint.

You have suffered a mild sprain involving a stretching of the ligaments.

With proper care it should start to feel better in about 3-4 days.

The healing process will be more effective if you follow this advice:

◆   Whenever possible, elevate the limb

◆   Continue to apply cold for 15 minute periods

◆   Remove the crepe roller bandage for sleeping

◆   You may notice some pain the following day when bearing weight with the crepe bandage removed. You may notice some increased swelling when the limb is not elevated

Report to first aid at the start of your next shift, the first aid attendant will reassess and re-bandage the injury if necessary.

You may need to discuss altering work activity with your supervisor.

If at any time you become unable to bear weight or the pain and swelling increase significantly, report to the first aid attendant, who may refer you to medical aid. If the condition becomes significantly worse while you are not at work, and you decide to seek medical aid, notify the first aid attendant as soon as possible.

Soft Tissue Injury to a Tendon (Tendonitis)

Tendonitis is the inflammation of the tendon.

You have tendonitis, also called RSI (repetitive strain injury) which is caused by excessive, unaccustomed activity.

With proper care it should start to feel better in about 3-4 days.

The healing process will be more effective by following this advice:

◆ Avoid motion that aggravates the tendons

◆ Keep the small splint in place as much as possible

◆ Continue to apply cold for 15 minute periods

◆ Alternating cold and heat may also assist in healing

◆ Remove the splint for sleeping

◆ You may notice minor pain the following day

◆ Report to first aid at the start of your next shift, the first aid attendant will reassess and reapply the splint if necessary

You may need to discuss altering work activity with your supervisor.

If at any time pain and swelling increase significantly, report to the first aid attendant, who may refer you to medical aid. If the condition becomes significantly worse while you are not at work and you decide to seek medical aid, notify the first aid attendant as soon as possible.

Flash Burns

Flash burns are burns to the surface of the cornea.

Direct or reflected ultraviolet light from an electric arc or welding torch may cause a flash burn. Corneal burns become more painful after some hours, depending on the severity and length of exposure.

Although flash burns are very uncomfortable, they are not serious and usually heal in 12-24 hours.

The healing process will be more effective by following this advice:

- Apply cold compresses at night for pain
- Avoid bright lights as this may aggravate the flash burns
- Wearing dark glasses may relieve some of the pain
- Mild pain medication (ASA or acetaminophen) may help to sleep at night
- You may notice minor pain the following day – this is normal
- Report to first aid at the start of your next shift
- The first aid attendant will reassess and document any symptoms you are experiencing

You may need to discuss altering work activity with your supervisor.

If at any time the pain increases significantly, report to the first aid attendant, who may refer you to medical aid. If the condition becomes significantly worse while you are not at work and you decide to seek medical aid, notify the attendant as soon as possible.

Minor Burns

You have a minor burn.

The reddening of you skin indicates a first degree burn. The presence of small blisters indicates a second degree burn.

The healing process will be more effective by following this advice:

- Keep the burned area covered
- Ensure the dressings stay dry and clean
- You may notice minor pain the following day – this is normal
- Report to first aid at the stat of your next shift
- The first aid attendant will reassess and document any symptoms you are experiencing

You may need to discuss altering work activity with your supervisor.

If at any time the pain increases significantly, report to the first aid attendant, who may refer you to medical aid. If the condition becomes significantly worse while you are not at work and you decide to seek medical aid, notify the attendant as soon as possible.

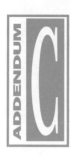

Legal Implications of First Aid in Alberta

Introduction

St. John Ambulance Emergency First Aid Safety Oriented (EFASO) for Industry with Alberta Endorsement -

- ◆ is recognized by the WorkSafe BC as equivalent to Occupational First Aid Level 1

- ◆ is approved by the Alberta Director of Medical Services for workplace Emergency Level First Aid training in Alberta

- ◆ meets Canada Labour Code requirements for Basic First Aid

On successful completion of the course, candidates will be issued a national St. John Ambulance Safety Oriented First Aid, Emergency Level certificate with Alberta Endorsement. The certificate is valid for two (2) years.

Alberta Emergency Medical Act

There are 3 Acts that an Alberta First Aider should be familiar with –

1. Emergency Medical Act
2. Alberta Occupational Health and Safety Act
3. Alberta Workers' Compensation Act

The Emergency Medical Act –

◆ is the name given to Alberta's Good Samaritan Laws

◆ protects first aiders from legal action providing they use reasonable skill and care and do not go beyond their level of training

◆ covers all of the points listed under the Good Samaritan Laws. First aiders must –

- act in good faith and volunteer their help
- tell the person they are trained in first aid
- get permission (consent) to give first aid before touching the casualty (consent is implied if the person is unresponsive)
- ask the parents or guardian for permission if the person is an infant or child
- use reasonable skill and care according to their level of training
- do not abandon (leave the person) once their offer of help has been accepted

Note: As long as first aiders follow the above principles and there is no obvious negligence, they should not be held liable.

Alberta Occupational Health & Safety Act

◆ is the umbrella legislation for all health and safety regulations for Alberta work sites.

◆ sets the standards to protect and promote the health and safety of workers

◆ encompasses –

(1) Occupational Health and Safety Code, and
(2) Occupational Health and Safety Regulation

Emergency Medical Act	Occupational Health and Safety Act		WCB Act
	OHS Code	**OHS Regulation**	**Section 37**
Protects first aiders from liability as long as they follow the principles and there is no obvious negligence. Under this act, first aiders must – ◆ act in good faith and volunteer their help ◆ tell the person they are trained in first aid ◆ get permission to give first aid before touching the casualty ◆ ask the parent or guardian for permission if the person is a child or infant ◆ do not abandon the person once their offer of help has been accepted.	**Part 4** Chemical and Biological Hazards and Harmful Substances **Part 11** First Aid **Part 29** WHMIS **Schedule 2: First Aid** **Table 1** Low Hazard Work **Table 2** High Hazard Work **Table 3** First Aid Equipment and Supplies **Table 4** First Aid Room Requirements **Table 5** First Aid Requirements for Low Hazard Work **Table 6** First Aid Requirements for Medium Hazard Work **Table 7** First Aid Requirements for High Hazard Work	Deals with administrative and policy issues	Requires workers and employers to report any workplace accident to the Workers' Compensation Board (WCB) where the injury disables or is likely to disable the worker beyond the day of the accident. Requires the employer to notify the WCB if the worker has had medical treatment or other services provided by licensed medical practitioners. Allows first aid records to be inspected by the WCB or a designate of the Board, and by the injured worker to whom the record(s) relates or to that worker's representative

Occupational Health and Safety Code

The OHS Code falls under the OHS Act. Alberta first aiders should be familiar with Part 4 (Section 27), **Part 11** (Sections 178-184), **Part 29** (Sections 407 and 413) **and Schedule 2** (Tables 1-7) **of the OHS Code.**

PART 4 **CHEMICAL & BIOLOGICAL HAZARDS & HARMFUL SUBSTANCES**

Section 27 Storage of harmful substances

- ◆ requires **employers** to clearly identify harmful substances at a work site even if they are exempt from WHMIS requirements.
- ◆ requires **employers** to store harmful substances in a safe manner

PART 11 **FIRST AID**

Section 178 Providing services, supplies, equipment

- ◆ requires **employers** to provide first aiders and have designated first aiders at work sites
- ◆ defines minimum standards in first aid services, equipment and supplies

Section 179 Location of first aid

- ◆ specifies the location and availability of first aid services, first aid equipment, supplies, and a first aid room (when necessary)
- ◆ specifies the maintenance and identification of first aid equipment and supplies
- ◆ requires the posting of signs indicating the location of first aid services, equipment and supplies
- ◆ requires a communication system be in place for workers to summon first aid services

Section 180 Emergency Transportation

- ◆ requires **employers** to ensure a means of transport is available for transporting injured or ill workers. If an ambulance is not available, then the means of transport must provide protection against the weather, have a means of communication with the health care facility, and be large enough to accommodate a stretcher and an accompanying person.

Section 181 First aid providers (See Schedule 2)

- ◆ states the employer's responsibility for ensuring the correct number and qualifications of first aiders at a work site

PART 11   FIRST AID

Section 182   Duties to report injury or illness

◆ requires **workers** to report illnesses or injuries that occur at work.

Section 183   Record of injury or illness

◆ requires the **employer** to record every acute illness or injury that occurs at the work site in a record kept for this purpose as soon as practicable after the illness or injury is reported to the employer.

◆ requires workplace **first aiders** to record work related injuries or sudden occurrences of illness that are reported to them. Information in the first aid record must include -

* employee name
* the date and time the illness or injury was reported
* a description of the acute illness or injury
* where the injury occurred
* the cause of the injury or acute illness
* first aid provided
* name of the first aider and level of first aid training

In the past, bound first aid treatment record books were kept in first aid kits and were available to anyone having access to the kits. In respecting worker privacy, the new First Aid Regulation limits access to first aid records and may prevent employees from continuing to use the bound treatment record books.

If first aid treatment records are kept in a first aid kit that all persons at the work site have access to, then single page forms should be used rather than books. Completed forms should be sent to an individual designated by the employer to keep all first aid records. Completed forms are not to be kept in the first aid kit.

Section 184   Access to first aid records

◆ requires that a person who has custody of records ensure that no person other than the worker has access to a worker's records unless the record is in a form that does not identify the worker or the worker has given written permission to the person, or the Director of Medical Services or a person authorized by the Director requires the records to be produced under the Act.

PART 29   WORKPLACE HAZARDOUS MATERIALS INFORMATION SYSTEM

Section 407   Availability of material safety data sheet

◆ requires **employers** to ensure that Material Safety Data Sheets(MSDSs) are available to workers who may be exposed to controlled products. **MSDSs include information on proper first aid treatment and can be a valuable resource for the workplace first aider.**

Section 413   Access to information by medical professionals

◆ gives medical personnel and first aiders access to information on controlled products (e.g. trade secrets) when necessary in order to diagnose or treat a worker.

SCHEDULE 2 FIRST AID TABLES 1-7

Table 1   Defines and specifies "low hazard work"

Table 2   Defines and specifies "High hazard work"

Table 3   Specifies first aid equipment and supplies contained in Number 1, Number 2, Number 3, and Type P first aid kits

Table 4   Specifies first aid room requirements

Table 5   Specifies first aid requirements for low hazard work based on (a) the number of workers at the work site per shift, and (b) the distance from the work site to medical aid

Table 6   Specifies first aid requirements for medium hazard work based on (a) the number of workers at the work site per shift, and (b) the distance from the work site to medical aid

Table 7   Specifies first aid requirements for high hazard work based on (a) the number of workers at the work site per shift, and (b) the distance from the work site to medical aid.

Occupational Health and Safety Regulations

Alberta's new Occupational Health and Safety regulation deals primarily with administrative and policy issues.

Alberta Workers' Compensation Act

Section 37   First Aid Records

◆ allows first aid records to be inspected by the WCB or a designate of the Board, and by the injured worker to whom the record(s) relates or to that worker's representative

Summary

ALBERTA EMERGENCY MEDICAL ACT

◆ is the name given to Alberta's Good Samaritan Law

◆ protects first aiders from legal action providing they use reasonable skill and care and do not go beyond their level of training

ALBERTA OCCUPATIONAL HEALTH AND SAFETY ACT

◆ is the umbrella legislation for all health and safety regulations for Alberta work sites

◆ encompasses the **(a) Occupational Health and Safety Code,** and **(b) Occupational Health and Safety Regulation**

a. Occupational Health and Safety Code
Part 4:
- Requires the employer to clearly identify harmful substances and store them in a safe manner

Part 11:
- Requires employers to provide first aiders at work sites
- Defines minimum standards for first aid services, equipment and supplies
- Requires a communication system for workers to summon first aid services
- Requires employers to ensure a means for transporting injured or ill workers
- Requires workers to report illnesses or injuries that occur at work
- Requires the employer to complete a first aid record for illnesses or injuries that occur at the work site
- Specifies who has access to first aid records
- Requires employers to ensure Material Safety Data Sheets are available to workers.

b. Occupational Health and Safety Regulation
- Deals primarily with administrative and policy issues

WORKERS COMPENSATION ACT

- allows **first aid records** to be inspected by the WCB, the injured worker, or his representative
- requires workers and employers to report workplace accidents to the WCB if the injury disables the worker beyond the day of the accident or if the worker requires medical treatment

ALBERTA FIRST AID RECORD

Date of injury or illness			Time		AM ☐
	Day	Month	Year		PM ☐

Date of injury or illness REPORTED			Time		AM ☐
	Day	Month	Year		PM ☐

Full name of injured or ill worker

Description of the injury or illness

Cause of injury or illness

First aid provided?   Yes ☐   No ☐   (If yes, complete the rest of this page)

Name of first aider:

First aider qualifications:

Emergency First Aider	☐	Emergency Medical Technician - Paramedic	☐
Standard First Aider	☐	Emergency Medical Techincian - Ambulance	☐
Advanced FIrst Aider	☐	Emergency Medical Technician	☐
Nurse	☐	Emergency Medical Responder	☐

First Aid provided:

Keep this record for at least 3 years from the date of injury or illness

Contact Information

Alberta Province-Wide Contact Centre

Edmonton	(780)415-8690
Other Locations in Alberta	1-866-415-8690

Deaf or Hearing Impaired

Edmonton	(780)427-9999
Other Locations in Alberta	1-800-232-7215

Getting Copies of OHS Act, Regulation and Code

Queen's Printer

Web Site: www.qp.gov.ab.ca

Edmonton (780)427-4952

Calgary (403)297-6251

Workplace Health and Safety

Web Site: www.whs.gov.ab.ca/law

Call any Government of Alberta office toll-free

Dial: 310-0000, then the area code and telephone number you want to reach

---

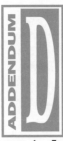

ADDENDUM D

Answer Key for Activities

Lesson 1 - Emergency Scene Management

1. First aid

2. a) preserve life

   b) prevent illness or injury from becoming worse

   c) promote recovery

3. Medical help

4. a) consent

   b) reasonable skill and care

   c) negligence

   d) abandonment

5. a) gloves

   b) face masks or shields

   c) hand washing

6. have

7. doesn't have

8. protect your own safety

9. Emergency Scene Management

10. a) scene survey

    b) primary survey

    c) secondary survey

    d) ongoing casualty care

11. a) airway

    b) breathing

    c) circulation

12. position found

13. a) medical help is delayed more than 20 minutes

    b) if you have to transport the casualty

    c) if the casualty has more than one injury

14. a) history of the casualty

    b) vital signs

    c) head-to-toe examination

    d) first aid for injuries found

15. a) give first aid for shock

    b) monitor the casualty's condition

    c) record the events of the situation

    d) report on what happened

16. take charge

    history

    head and neck

    medical help

    should not

    a) what happened

    b) what kind of injuries are involved

    c) what first aid has been given

Lesson 2 - Shock

1. Shock

   unconsciousness, death

2. a) severe burns

   b) crush injuries

   c) heart attack

   d) spinal cord injuries

   e) severe allergic reactions

3. *any four from the list on page 2-2*

4. the casualty's condition

5. a) give first aid for injuries or illness

   b) reassure the casualty often

   c) handle the casualty gently

   d) loosen tight clothing at the neck, chest and waist

   e) keep casualty warm

   f) moisten llips but do not give anything to drink

   g) place the casualty in the best position possible for their condition

   h) continue ongoing care until hand over

6. medical, medical help

7. a) eye opening response

   b) verbal response

   c) motor response

8. recovery

9. loss of consciousness

10. pale

    sweating

    feels sick, nauseous, dizzy and unsteady

D-1

11. lying down

feet raised

12. unconsciousness

Lesson 3 - Choking - Adult

1. should not

2. inward, upward

3. a) the object is removed

b) the person becomes unconscious

4. will not

medical help

5. medical help

6. breathe

7. chest compressions

8. should

9. chest

10. lose consciousness

11. a) your hands

b) a piece of furniture - e.g. chair

Lesson 4 - Cardiovascular emergencies - CPR

1. Cardiovascular disease

2. fatty deposits

oxygen

3. Angina

4. medication

5. heart attack

6. *any four from the list on page 4-4*

7. medical help

8. a) at rest

b) prescribed medication

c) CPR

9. stroke or cerebrovascular accident (CVA)

10. transient ischemic attack (or TIA)

11. stroke

12. *any four from the list on page 4-7*

13 artificial respiration

chest compressions

14. medical help

AED

15. 30

2

four from the list in step 10 on page 4-13

Lesson 5 - Severe Bleeding

1. dressing

2. a) hold a dressing in place

b) maintain pressure over a wound

c) support a limb or joint

d) immobilize parts of the body

e) secure a splint

3. triangular

a) whole cloth

b) broad bandage

c) narrow bandage

d) ring pad

4. *some examples are shown on page 5-5 but most anything that with the appropriate characteristics is acceptable here*

5. a) direct pressure

b) rest

6. circulation

7. a) control bleeding

b) care for amputated tissue

c) get medical help

8. a) becomes more painful

b) becomes red and perhaps swollen

c) feels warmer than surrounding area

d) shows the presence of pus

9. Tetanus

10. *any three of the six from the list on page 5-13*

11. blood is

a) coming from ear canal, nose, eyes

b) coughed up or looks bright red

c) seen in vomitus

d) seen in stools

e) seen in urine

12. shock (on their back with feet and legs raised)

recovery

13. medical help

Lesson 6 - Medical conditions

1. insulin

2.   Diabetes

3.   *any four from the chart on page 6-2*

4.   *any four from the chart on page 6-2*

5.   medical alert device

6.   sugar

      juice

7.   seizure

8.   a) don't restrict the casualty's
      movements

      b) carefully loosen tight clothing

      c) place something soft under the head

      d) do not try to put anything in the
      mouth

9.   *any two from the list on page 6-4*

10.   a) protect the child from injury

      b) loosen tight clothing

11.   Asthma

12.   *any four from the list on page 6-7*

13.   a) pet hair

      b) pollen, paint and smoke

      c) certain foods

      d) insect bites or stings

14.   metered-dose inhaler

15.   anaphylaxis

16.   *any four from the list on page 6-9*

17.   auto-injector

18.   medical help

Lesson 15 (BC) - Minor Wound Care

2.   a) Split open wound to the palm of the
      hand that is difficult to close

      b) Deep wound over a knuckle

      c) Wound caused by a rusty nail that is
      lodged in the tissue

4.   c) Control bleeding and prevent infection

6.   a) False

      b) True

      c) True

      d) False

8.   b) Clean small wounds before aplpying a
      dressing

      c) Wipe away from the wound with a
      clean price of gauze or remove dirt

10.   a) Before and after bandaging a wound
      to a limb

      c) For all major and minor wounds to
      limbs

12.   a) Choice 2

      b) Choice 1

14.   a) False

      b) True

      c) True

      d) False

16.   a) True

      b) False

      c) True

      d) True

18.   a) True

      b) False

      c) True

      d) True

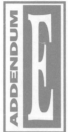

FIRST AID EXAMINATION ANSWER SHEET
Emergency First Aid Safety Oriented PLEASE PRINT

Student's Name: _____ Date: _____

Provincial Council/Special Centre: _____

Final marks: Section 1: ____ *(Pass = 18/25)* Section 2: ____ *(Pass = 4/5)*

1 ✔
Section 1:
EFASO

1.	a	b	c	d
2.	a	b	c	d
3.	a	b	c	d
4.	a	b	c	d
5.	a	b	c	d
6.	a	b	c	d
7.	a	b	c	d
8.	a	b	c	d
9.	a	b	c	d
10.	a	b	c	d
11.	a	b	c	d
12.	a	b	c	d
13.	a	b	c	d
14.	a	b	c	d
15.	a	b	c	d
16.	a	b	c	d
17.	a	b	c	d
18.	a	b	c	d
19.	a	b	c	d
20.	a	b	c	d
21.	a	b	c	d
22.	a	b	c	d
23.	a	b	c	d
24.	a	b	c	d
25.	a	b	c	d

2
Section 2:
Alberta Endorsement

26.	a	b	c	d
27.	a	b	c	d
28.	a	b	c	d
29.	a	b	c	d
30.	a	b	c	d

WHAT NEXT?!

Congratulations!

You have successfully completed a St. John Ambulance First Aid course. What next?

Why not put your new skills to use, and become a volunteer member of St. John Ambulance?

Join our Community Services Programs

▶ **serve your community** — provide first aid services at local events, or take part in other programs such as our Therapy Dog Program.

▶ **learn more first aid, CPR and patient care skills**—ongoing training for members integrates first aid, CPR and patient care skills along with practical and written assessments.

▶ **develop leadership skills**—take advantage of leadership training and apply it within our programs.

▶ **make new friends**—there are over 500 local units across the country, made up of over 12,000 people, like yourself, who want to share their time and skills with their communities.

▶ **earn recognition**—your involvement in Community Services programs will be appreciated by the community you serve. Your achievements will be recognized through our awards program.

Become an Instructor

▶ **teach courses to the public**—further your knowledge and techniques through the Instructor Certification Program, and share your talents through community-based courses.

▶ **earn an honorarium**—expenses incurred while teaching classes will be covered by an honorarium.

▶ **help Canadians to help themselves**—with your help, Canadians will learn new skills in the variety of courses offered by St. John Ambulance.

▶ **gain experience speaking in front of a group**—you will have an opportunity to speak to Canadians young and old, and from a variety of cultural backgrounds. Each new group offers new and different challenges.

▶ **develop lasting friendships**—participating as a St. John instructor can lead to developing friendships with your fellow instructors.

Share your skills—join the St. John family.

For more information, contact your local St. John Ambulance office today!

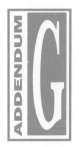

ADDENDUM **G**

Type of Course:	First aid
	Emergency Level ☐ Standard Level ☐
	CPR (please indicate which level) ———————
	AED ☐

Please print all information clearly.

STUDENT'S NAME (As you want it to appear on your certificate.)

FIRST NAME Martin	MIDDLE INITIAL L	LAST NAME Hallat

APT/STREET/P.O. BOX 5390 Wallace Ave.	HOME TELEPHONE (INCLUDING AREA CODE) 604-943-4064

CITY/TOWN Delta	PROVINCE BC	POSTAL CODE V4M 1H1

E-MAIL ADDRESS generalhallat@hotmail.com	DATE OF BIRTH (OPTIONAL)

( ) I agree to abide by the principles of first aid and the terms and conditions as outlined in the

EFASO Student Reference Guide. _____ (Signature of Applicant)

EMPLOYER INFORMATION

COMPANY/ORGANIZATION BC Ferries	EMPLOYEE NO. 101259

APT/STREET/P.O. BOX #1 Ferry Causeway	FAX 604-943-3028

CITY/TOWN Delta	WORK TELEPHONE (INCLUDING AREA CODE) 604-943-9331

PROVINCE BC	POSTAL CODE V4M 4G6	E-MAIL

Thank you for taking a course with St. John Ambulance and helping us to meet our goal of:

"training one person in each household in first aid and CPR"

If you enjoyed the course, and felt it was valuable to your workplace, home or family, why not put your skills to use and become a volunteer or instructor with St. John Ambulance. Please identify your interest by checking the following:

☐ I am interested in becoming:
☐ a volunteer member with St. John Ambulance or
☐ an instructor with St. John Ambulance

See Addendum F for additional information or visit www.sja.ca

☐ I am interested in subscribing to receive additional information about St. John Ambulance, including subscription to our online newsletter, surveys, and the like. It is acknowledged and recognized that in some instances, St. John Ambulance partners or sponsors may provide subscribers with additional promotion material. As in all cases, St. John Ambulance will not rent, sell or lease your information to a third party.

Privacy Statement

The information collected is for the purpose of verifying student name, mailing address for delivery of certification, and for student's to opt-in to receiving volunteer, instructor, and/or promotional information. Information is retained for the certification period of the certificate, to provide notification of recertification, and/or for the receipt of additional information requested. For further information regarding St. John Ambulance's privacy statement for students, please visit www.sja.ca